homespa

BODY MIND SPIRIT

JENNIE HARDING

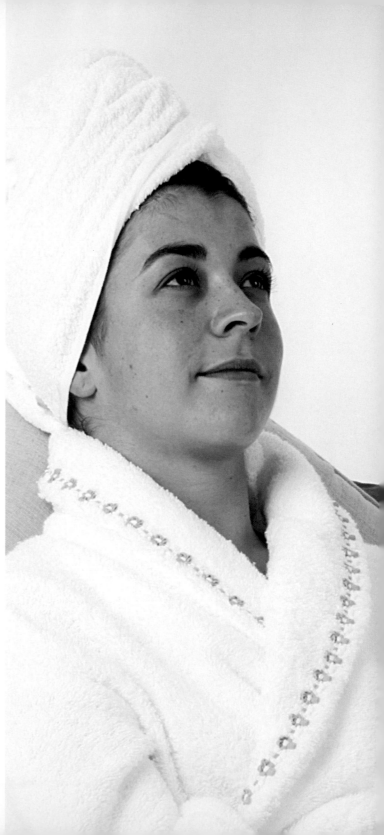

This is a Parragon Book
This edition published in 2006

Parragon
Queen Street House
4 Queen Street Bath
BA1 1HE UK

ISBN: 1-40546-382-1

Printed in China

Produced by the Bridgewater Book Company Ltd

Photographer: Calvey Taylor-Haw

PICTURE CREDITS:

Corbis: p.5, 63 & 103 Stephen Welstead; p.6 Rob Lewine;
p.7 & 87 Jutta Klee; p.9 & 107 Michael Keller; p.23 Dann Tardif;
p.24, 31 Larry Williams; p.44 Ariel Skelley; p.54 Layne Kennedy;
p.56 Mark M. Lawrence; p.61 Joaquin Palting; p.68 Walter Smith;
p.91 Chris Hellier; p.94 Richard T. Nowitz; p.104 Rick Gomez;
p.105 Jim Cummins.

This book is dedicated to Rosie and Bill with love and thanks.

CONTENTS

INTRODUCTION

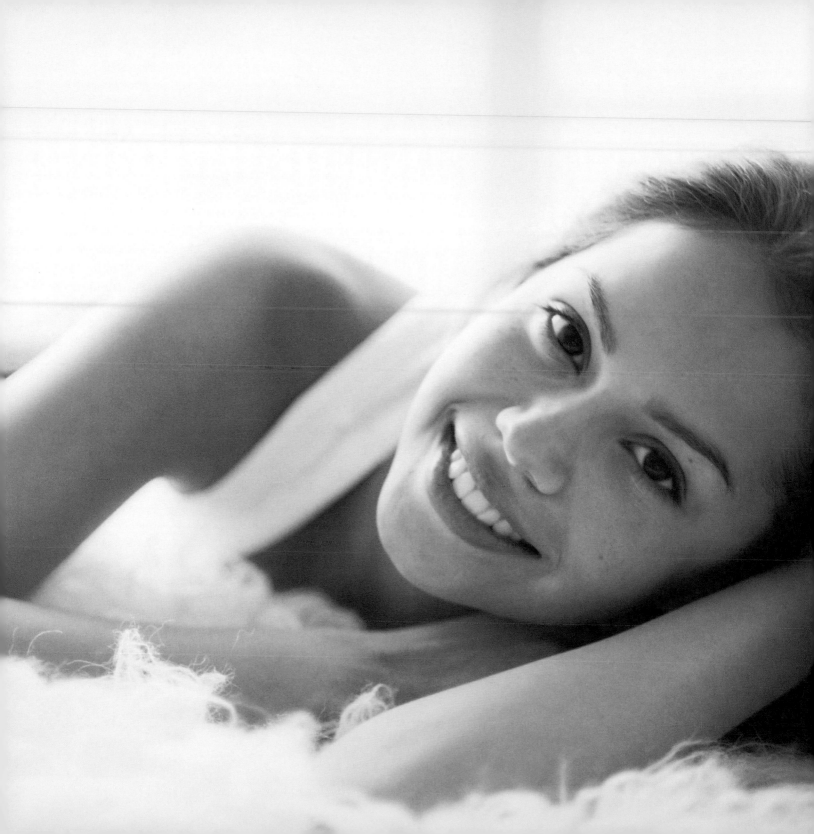

WHY CREATE YOUR OWN SPA?

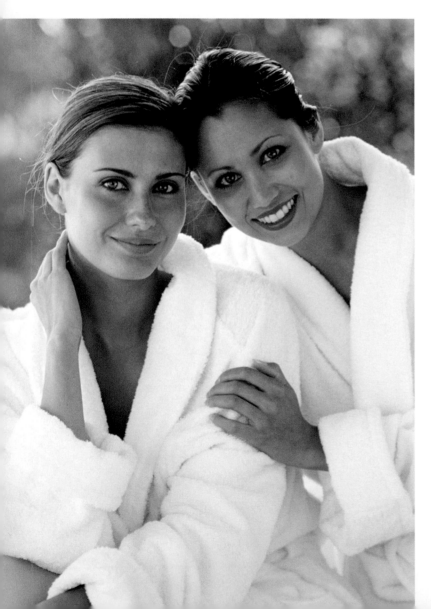

How often do you really take time out? As we try to cram more work and activities into our lives, it is important to stop sometimes, although this usually doesn't happen often enough. Going to a gym can be a way of unwinding, but exercise can often increase feelings of tiredness, especially if you don't include some relaxation time afterwards. Exercise and relaxation need to be in balance so that they can assist your body to recover from the challenges of everyday life.

In a spa – a place providing health-giving treatments, exercise and relaxation – this balance can easily be experienced. A spa is a place of retreat where you can choose from a range of activities to create a balance between effort and rest. Both of these aspects are vital to your body. Effort through exercise builds muscle and stamina, while rest and relaxation allow repair and rejuvenation.

Different spa treatments help to cleanse and revitalize body and mind. The use of water – **HYDROTHERAPY** – cleanses the skin, stimulates blood flow and assists the body to detoxify itself.

Various types of massage – **BODY THERAPY** – ease out physical tensions and assist the body's process of repair. Outdoor exercise is particularly recommended as a way of filling the lungs with rejuvenating oxygen. Finally, cleansing foods and drinks are provided – **DIETARY THERAPY** – to cleanse the system from inside.

The role of nature in the process of cleansing is vital, feeding all the senses – sight, hearing, touch, taste and smell – and bringing a sense of peace and tranquillity. For this reason, many famous spas are situated in beautiful countryside, in mountain scenery or by the sea. A spa is one of the most holistic ways of treating your whole self to a true and complete rest.

Since for many of us a trip to a spa is unaffordable, in either time or money, this book, **HOME SPA: BODY, MIND, SPIRIT**, will show you how to create a spa setting in your own home. Learn to give yourself, your partner and your friends the experience of natural spa treatments, have fun making your own spa recipes and take time out to nurture and pamper yourself the home spa way.

SAFETY – though all ingredients used in this book are natural, it is still important to follow the safety tips on page 17.

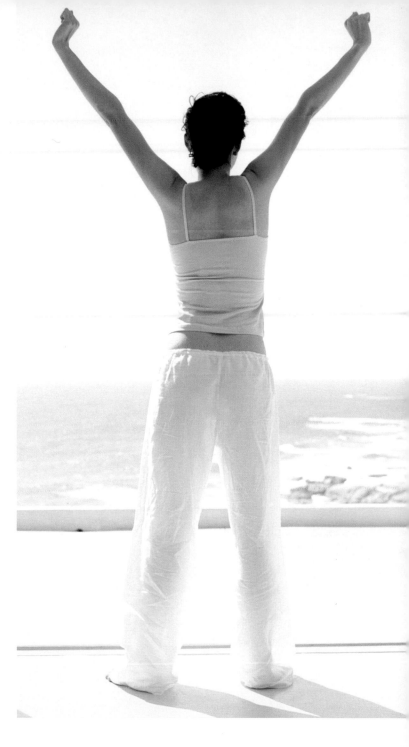

HOW TO HAVE FUN WITH A HOME SPA

You don't have to live in a mansion, or even have a garden, to create a spa environment in your home. Parks or open spaces near your home can give you access to nature, balconies can be used for resting and windows opened to let in air. You don't need complicated equipment either: all the recipes for foods, drinks and treatments can easily be made in your kitchen, and the water treatments just need your bathroom. The only other thing you need is space to rest and receive body treatments – for which a sitting room or bedroom is perfect. A home spa helps you to treat yourself in the comfort of a familiar space.

CREATE YOUR OWN HOME SPA

IT'S SIMPLE With a bit of organization and planning, you will be surprised at how easily you can create 'spa time' for yourself, for you and a friend or partner, or for a group of people. The marvellous thing about it is that it feels such a treat; it is fun to share or simply to give a home spa to yourself.

IT'S FLEXIBLE In this book you will find lots of different home spa routines – some as short as 30 minutes – so anyone can fit 'spa time' into a busy schedule. I guarantee that the taster sessions will make you want more, and you will find two-hour, one-day and even whole weekend programmes in the following chapters, so you can really pick and choose. The spa routines can also work alongside your existing exercise pattern.

IT'S NATURALLY GOOD FOR YOU All the recipes for home spa treatments use 100 per cent natural ingredients, and the superb cleansers, toners, nourishers and soothers, which lavish care on your skin, are totally free of harsh chemicals. The ingredients are very easy to source, then all you need are spoons, bowls and normal kitchen equipment to mix and prepare them – including a refrigerator to keep things cool – and you're ready to start the treatments.

BODY TREATMENT
SOME OF THE RECIPES TO LOOK FORWARD TO:
Cardamom & Grapefruit Aromatherapy Skin Blend
Oatmeal, Yogurt & Geranium Face Mask
Sugar & Lemon Exfoliating Scrub
Peppermint & Rosemary Nourishing Body Scrub

You'll also find delicious juices, smoothies and healthy treats to enjoy during home spa time, such as:
Banana & Orange Smoothie
Papaya & Raspberry Whirl

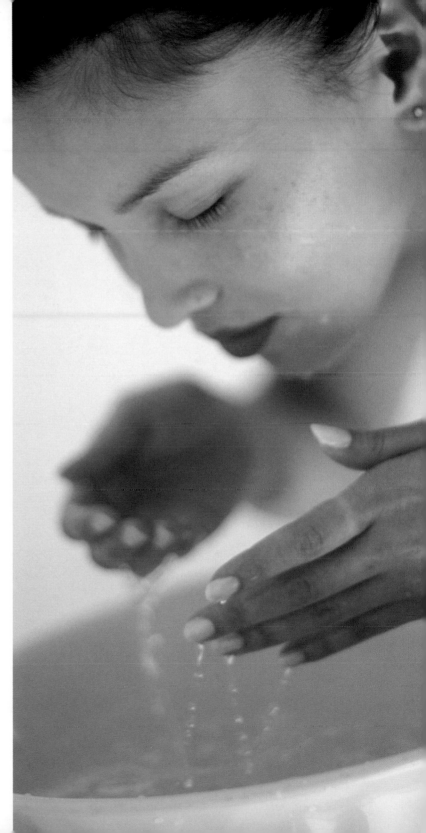

CHAPTER ONE

WHAT YOU WILL NEED

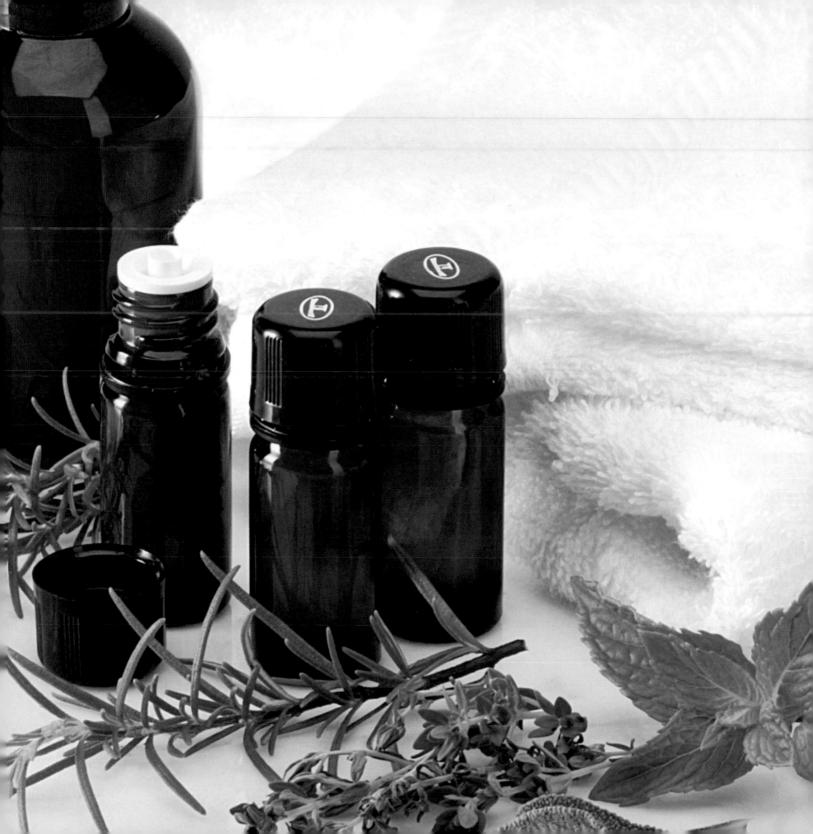

PREPARING YOUR HOME SPA

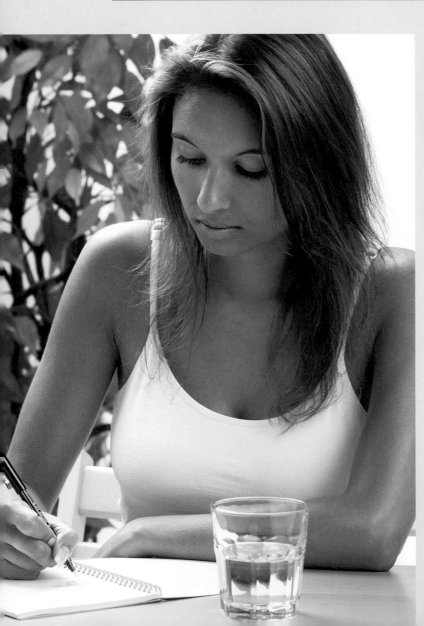

Your home spa will need to be organized, but this can be part of the fun and anticipation of the time you will spend pampering and caring for yourself. See it all as part of the process of creating a healthy, happy and energized new you. Home spa time will encourage you to make health care part of your everyday life, especially if you do it regularly. Listed below are some of the key elements you will need to think about.

TIME

How much time do you want to give yourself? That means time away from distractions – including the phone and the TV. Home spa time means total retreat – putting on the answerphone, switching off your mobile, and telling your family not to disturb you for a specified time. Isolating yourself in this way is the biggest challenge when using your own home, and you need to be firm about it. If you are very busy, start with one of the short routines in Chapter 2; once you have tried a few of these, you may then be ready to move on to the weekend home spa session in Chapter 3.

PLANNING

Think ahead – and be creative. Check your diary; if you are choosing one of the routines in Chapter 2, these will fit into an evening or a day off. The full weekend routine in Chapter 3 could be used to start off a holiday period – or you could use it to chill out with a friend or partner after a busy week at work. In Chapters 2 and 3 you will find 'menus' for your chosen programmes with suggested lists of ingredients you will need. It's best to get everything together in advance so that you don't have to dash to the supermarket in the middle of it all.

WATER

This is your inner cleanser. Water is crucial in a home spa, both for hydrotherapy and for internal cleansing. You need to drink at least 8 large glasses of water during a one-day programme, so it is very important to have plentiful supplies of mineral water on hand. If you don't like drinking water on its own, for the home spa experience buy yourself a beautiful glass to drink it from – it really does make a difference – and make sure the water is deliciously chilled. Water should be drunk plain, without slices of lemon, to give your kidneys the full detoxifying benefit.

SETTING UP YOUR SPACE

Your home is going to be used in a very different way during a home spa, so you need to get it ready. This is a space-clearing exercise to be done as part of your preparation; you will notice that the energy of your home improves even before you begin your home spa time, changing from 'normal' to 'special'. Use the ideas outlined below.

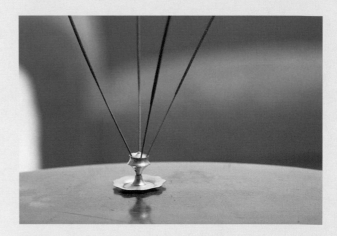

TIDYING AND CLEANING

Yes, it's a chore, but remember – this is all for your benefit. Go through your home spa space thoroughly and clear up piles of newspapers, magazines and other clutter; shake cushions, straighten throws over the sofa and give the carpet a good vacuum; dust window sills and open curtains to let in light; finally, open windows to let in fresh air. In the kitchen, tidy and clean and make sure that all the ingredients that need cold storage are in the refrigerator. Prepare the bathroom and place candles in dishes to burn while you soak in the water.

INCENSE

This purifies the air once the space is clean. There are 2 forms – stick incense needs to be secured in a suitable holder, while incense in cones can be placed on a saucer. Indian incense tends to have a sandalwood or patchouli base and smells sweet and musky; Tibetan incense often has a more earthy, forest-like aroma. Finally, Native American incense has a pine or sage aroma with a fresh, bracing effect.

FLOWERS

Fresh flowers brought into your space in lovely vases create colour, shapes and aromas: they immediately bring the beauty of nature inside. If you have a garden, you may like to select flowers you grow yourself and create your own displays; otherwise you could buy a selection and arrange them.

TEMPERATURE

This needs to be set so that the atmosphere is warm and comfortable. In autumn or winter, this will mean turning up the central heating, because you will be dressed in a robe or towels for much of the time. In spring or summer, the important thing is to ventilate your space so that it is comfortable inside, depending on the weather.

MUSIC

Have a sound system available to play relaxing and inspiring music while you enjoy your spa sessions. Choose music that is soothing, such as classical or gentle 'New Age' music with natural sounds. World music, such as Tibetan chanting or gong playing, is also very restful.

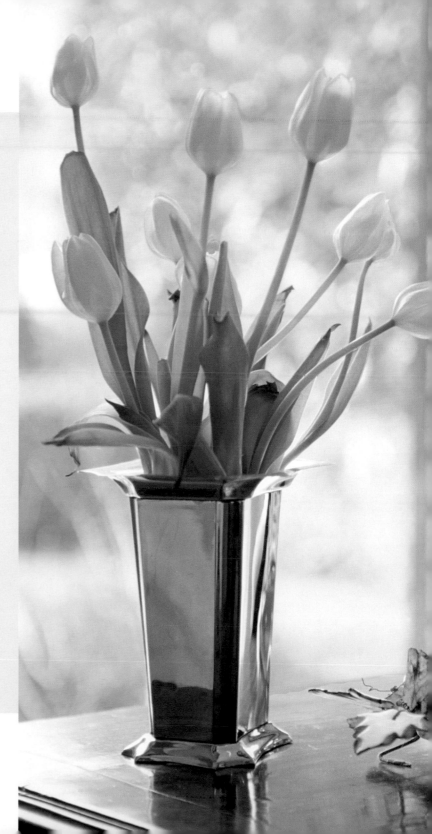

SIMPLE AROMATHERAPY

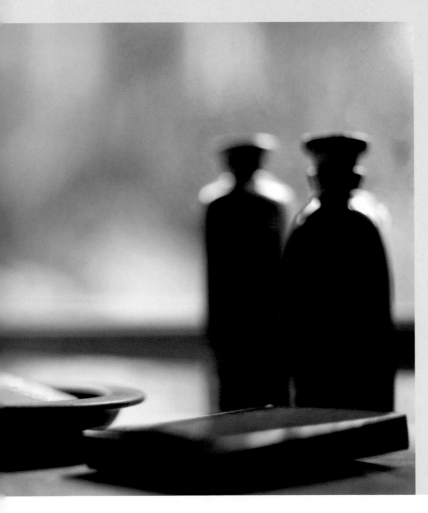

Aromatherapy is one of the tools used in the home spa setting. It uses special natural plant extracts, called essential oils, to create wonderful fragrances with beneficial effects on body and mind. Eight key essential oils have been chosen for the home spa kit, to be used in massage blends, in the bath and in facial steaming. Here the oils are introduced along with simple aromatherapy information and methods; for more detail on each individual oil, see pages 90–1.

OIL	HOME SPA USE
CARDAMOM	stimulating, warming, pain relieving
CYPRESS	skin toning, cleansing, balancing
GERANIUM	skin hydrating, soothing, nourishing
GRAPEFRUIT	cleansing, detoxifying, stimulating
JUNIPER	detoxifying, stimulating, warming
LAVENDER	soothing, skin rejuvenating, pain relieving
LEMON	cleansing, antiseptic, toning
YLANG YLANG	skin hydrating, balancing, rejuvenating

METHODS

MAKING A BLEND Take a small clean bowl. Measure 4 teaspoons carrier oil into it. Add your essential oil drops as per the recipe, stir, and the blend is ready to use.

BATHS Run the bath to a comfortable temperature, add drops of oil to a carrier, e.g. milk, as per the recipe, and swish into the water before getting in.

FACIAL STEAMING Pour near-boiling water into a heatproof glass bowl so that it is two-thirds full. Add drops of essential oil to the surface as per the recipe, lean over the bowl with your head under a towel so the steam reaches your skin, and stay there for 15 minutes.

STORING ESSENTIAL OILS

Once you open bottles of these essential oils, grapefruit and lemon will last for 6 months only, while the other 6 will last for up to 1 year. Keep them in the dark, tightly closed.

SAFETY TIPS

1 If you are pregnant, avoid juniper in any blends or bath recipes. Substitute with lavender instead. Drops of essential oil in any given recipes must be halved in the same amount of carrier oil or base, or halved for the bath.

2 If you apply a blend using either grapefruit or lemon oil in massage, avoid exposing the skin to strong sunlight or a sunbed for 12 hours after application.

3 Never swallow essential oils; use them only on the skin, in the bath or as a steam treatment. Keep out of the reach of children.

4 Always purchase essential oils in dark glass bottles with dropper inserts in the neck to dispense 1 drop at a time.

5 Never let any of the preparations get in your eyes. If this should happen, rinse immediately with warm water.

6 All the recipes are for 1 application only, unless they are made for treatments to be shared with a partner. Do not store any of the preparations, but use immediately, unless otherwise stated.

SIMPLE HERBS

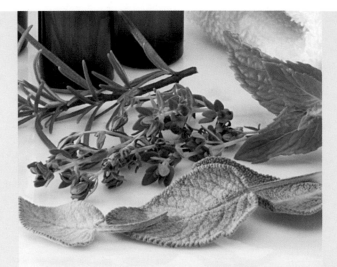

Herbs are very important in the spa setting. All over the world, people of different cultures use their indigenous plants to support the health of the skin as well as the body. Mediterranean herbs are very easy to obtain and are renowned for their toning and soothing properties. They are particularly useful in the spa setting in baths and in steam treatments, as well as foot baths. Many can be obtained fresh all year round; they can also be used dried. Eight key herbs feature in the home spa kit; they are introduced here along with simple herbal methods. For more information on individual herbs, see pages 92–3.

WATER INFUSIONS (TEAS)

Place 1 teaspoon dried herbs or 2 teaspoons freshly chopped leaves/flowers in a mug. Then pour over 100 ml/3.5 fl oz near-boiling water, place a saucer over the mug and leave to infuse for 15 minutes. Hot infusions can be drunk to help digestion and inner cleansing; cold infusions can be used as skin fresheners or hair rinses. They need to be used on the day of brewing.

BATHS

If you are using dried herbs, it is best to place them in a small muslin bag, which you tie over the tap as the water runs in; use 3 teaspoons per bath. If you are using fresh herbs, simply gather a handful of fresh leaves or flowers and scatter them over the surface of the water.

FACIAL STEAMING

Pour near-boiling water into a heatproof bowl so that it is two-thirds full. If you are using a dried herb, add 1 teaspoon to the water; if you are using a fresh herb, add 2 teaspoons freshly chopped leaves or flowers to the water. Lean over the bowl into the steam with your head under a towel; stay there for 15 minutes.

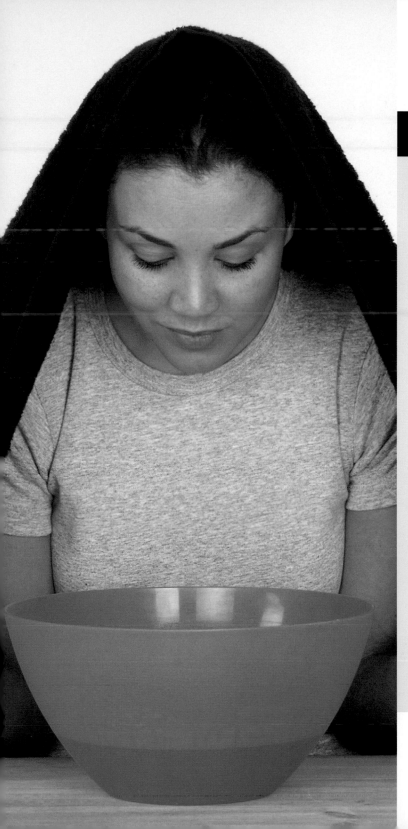

BENEFITS OF USING HERBS

HERB	HOME SPA USE
MELISSA [LEMON BALM]	skin soothing, calming, restorative
MYRTLE	skin soothing, rejuvenating, refreshing
PEPPERMINT	toning, cleansing, refreshing
ROMAN CHAMOMILE	skin soothing, calming, anti-inflammatory
ROSEMARY	stimulating, warming, pain relieving
SAGE	toning, fortifying, cleansing
SWEET MARJORAM	skin soothing, restorative, calming
THYME	cleansing, refreshing, skin toning

SIMPLE HERB SAFETY

Do not exceed the stated amounts in recipes. Herbal teas, baths and skin preparations are safe to use during pregnancy, but do not use the same herb for more than 3 days at a time without consulting a qualified practitioner.

HOME SPA EQUIPMENT

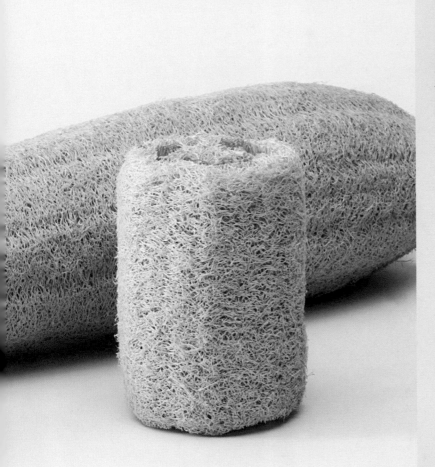

Although it is not necessary to have complicated equipment for a home spa, there are some items that do increase the effectiveness of skin treatments. This is particularly important when you want to stimulate the detoxification process. It is easy to find these items in stores that specialize in health products. You do not need to have them all – a selection is enough. The following are some of the items you might want to buy.

LOOFAH

This is a natural sea gourd with a rough texture that softens when you wet it. It is used to stimulate the circulation in the shower; rub your shower gel or body scrub on to the skin and use the loofah in circular motions to create a skin-warming effect.

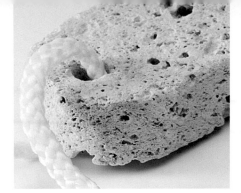

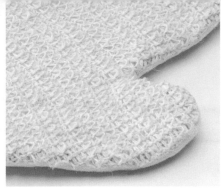

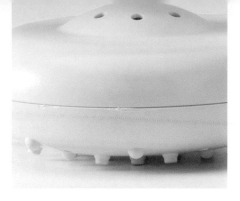

PUMICE STONE

This is a soft grey stone of volcanic origin that helps to remove calloused or very dry skin from the heels in particular. It is important to soak the feet before using it, and to massage the heels gently; always apply a rich moisturizer to follow.

FRICTION GLOVE

Often made from coarse material, this glove helps to stimulate the circulation and can be used in the bath or shower, particularly on problem areas such as the thighs or underarms. It should be used in circular motions, starting gently, and with care on sensitive skin.

CELLULITE MASSAGER

This rounded massage aid has rubber nodules on its lower surface, which help to stimulate the deeper tissue beneath the upper skin layers. It can be used with a shower gel or scrub, or with an aromatherapy massage blend, and is most often used on the thighs.

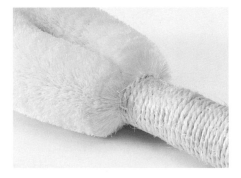

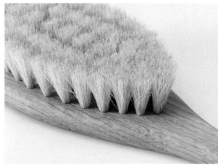

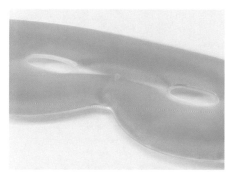

SKIN BRUSH

This soft brush is used on dry skin before a bath or shower treatment. It is particularly good for cold hands and feet. Start at the ends of the fingers and toes and brush up towards the heart in circular sweeps.

BACK BRUSH

This long-handled brush is useful to reach the back when you are in the bath; it can also be used on solo spa days to apply body scrub, improving the circulation and skin condition of areas that are hard to reach.

COOLING EYE MASK

This is a mask filled with gel, which you place in the refrigerator for at least an hour before laying it over the eye area. It reduces puffiness and helps you to relax your eyes, easing mental tension.

CHAPTER TWO

SIMPLE HOME SPA ROUTINES

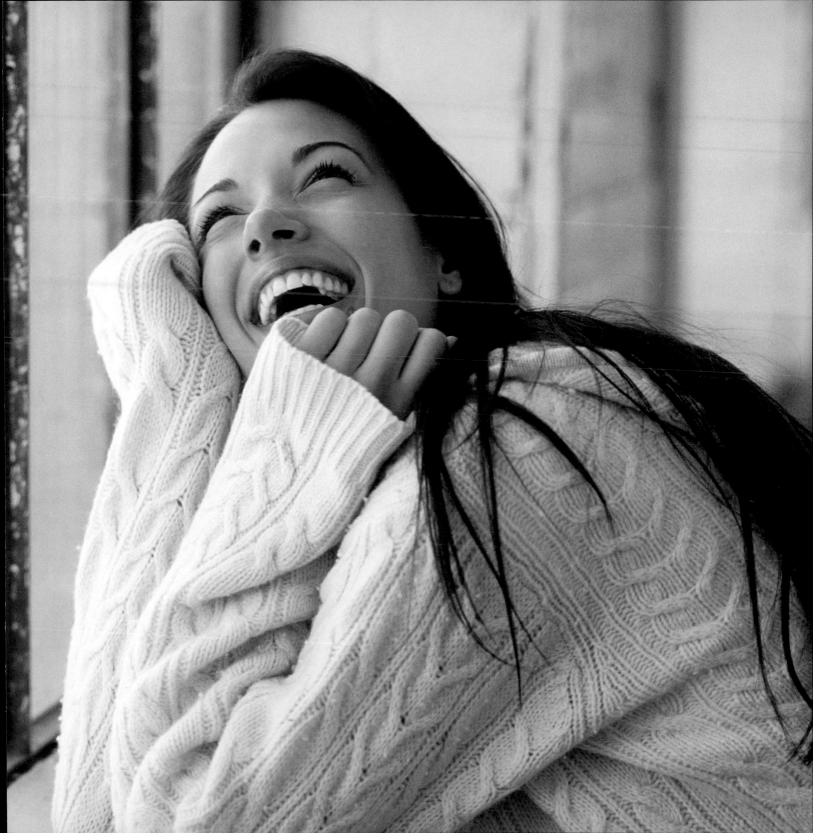

HOME SPA TIME TO
SUIT YOUR LIFESTYLE

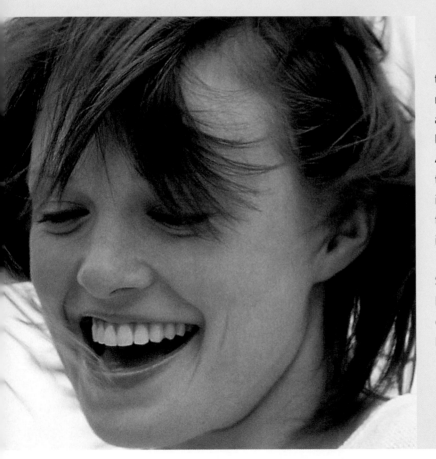

In the following pages you will find 4 different short routines that are designed to fit into anyone's schedule – no matter how busy they are. They range from just a simple shower routine right through to one-day programmes, and all are packed with lush ingredients and lovely recipes to try. Here is an overview of all 4 routines to give you an idea of their content; this should make it easy to choose which one is right for you. Once you have decided, go to the relevant pages and you will find all the instructions you need to get started.

Spa treatments are a great way to keep fit and healthy. However, if you have a recognized medical condition, please consult your doctor before beginning your spa.

ROUTINE 1: Wake Up and Go in 30 Minutes [see pages 26–9]

Turn your shower into a mini-spa session that's short enough to fit into your early morning routine but also effective at boosting your energy. Use a special shower scrub to invigorate your skin, and give yourself an in-shower acupressure scalp massage.

ROUTINE 2: Girlie Spa Day [see pages 30–43]

Enjoy a special fun day designed for a group of girls who want to spend a healthy day pampering each other with gorgeous natural foot, face and hand treatments. Try it for a pre-wedding celebration or as a special treat for someone's birthday.

ROUTINE 3: Solo Spa Day [see pages 44–53]

This is a lovely calm, relaxing day programme that enables you to unwind by yourself. This programme is a treat to the senses, with a detoxifying bath, rich massage blends and a lavish full facial treatment designed to give you a sense of deep tranquillity.

ROUTINE 4: Two-hour Evening Spa [see pages 54–61]

This easy session, which uplifts the spirits and refreshes the mind, is a wonderful way to recover at the end of a demanding day. Try a hot oil hair treatment, a special detox shower and a wonderful neck and shoulder massage, with essential oils and herbs to create wonderful aromas all around you.

REFRESH WITH WATER

All these routines are combined with special suggestions for healthy foods, drinks and treats – cleansing you from inside out.

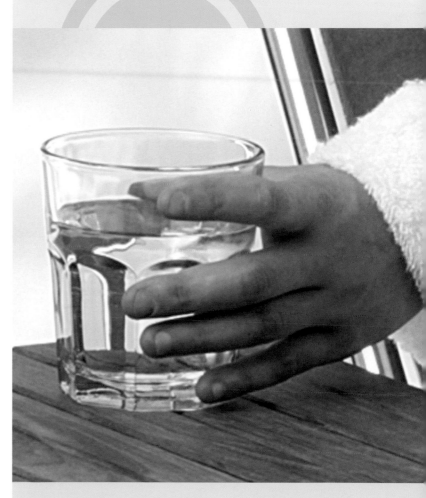

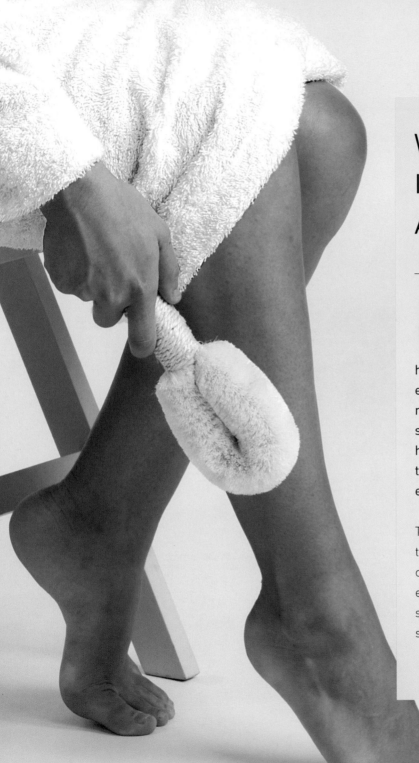

WAKE UP AND GO IN 30 MINUTES: A MINI SPA

C an you have a spa in 30 minutes? Yes, you can. This is a really quick and easy session that makes your shower work harder for you, deep-cleansing your skin and energizing your whole body through a scalp massage. If you don't have a shower, you can still do this routine in a bath, washing your hair in the water; just make sure that the temperature is not too hot – you want to be energized, not boiled.

The combination of skin rub and exfoliating treatment on these pages helps to stimulate the circulation immediately under the skin, which then encourages the removal of toxins through your system. Have a large glass of water after the shower to encourage elimination.

WAKE UP AND GO MENU

Make up the recipes in advance.

TREATMENTS

Dry skin pre-shower brush [see opposite]
Shower with Grapefruit & Sea Salt Body
    Scrub [see opposite]
In-shower scalp massage [see page 28]
All-over body massage with Cardamom
    & Grapefruit Aromatherapy Skin Blend
    [see page 29]

DRINK: Banana & Orange Smoothie, full of
vitamins for energy [see page 29]

INGREDIENTS

dry skin brush	grapeseed carrier oil
fine sea salt	1 banana
grapefruit and cardamom	1 orange
essential oils	natural yogurt

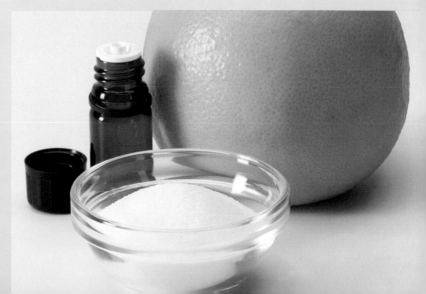

● ● ● ○ TREATMENT ADVICE

Use home spa treatments on the day of making.
Avoid contact with the eyes. If the treatment
gets into the eyes, rinse well with warm water.

PART 1

DRY SKIN BRUSHING

First, prepare your skin for the shower using a dry skin brush. The soft bristles gently stimulate and wake up your circulation. Start at the feet and make small circular motions over the toes and up the legs, towards the hips; then start at the fingertips and make circles up towards the heart. Then get in the shower and lather the skin with a good quality shower gel.

GRAPEFRUIT & SEA SALT BODY SCRUB

Place 3 tablespoons fine sea salt in a small bowl; add 6 drops grapefruit essential oil and stir in. Get in the shower but do not turn the water on yet. Take a handful of the mixture and rub it briskly all over your body, especially your thighs and stomach. Rinse off the skin well. Grapefruit is cleansing and detoxifying, and the sea salt is an excellent exfoliator, removing loose dead cells and leaving the skin glowing and ready for moisturizing.

PART 2

The second part of the in-shower mini-spa routine involves a special simple acupressure massage to the scalp. This is very useful to help wake you up physically as well as mentally. The scalp is covered with acupressure points, which stimulate energy through the meridians (the energy lines that run throughout the body). When you have dried yourself, you can then apply a nourishing but non-greasy essential oil blend, which will pamper your skin beautifully during the day. Finally, whizz up and drink a delicious, vitamin-packed Banana & Orange Smoothie.

IN-SHOWER SCALP MASSAGE

Lather your hair with a nourishing shampoo; then, while the shampoo is still on your hair, place both hands on either side of your head with your fingers above your ears. Apply pressure in tiny, firm, circular movements with all your fingertips, then move up slightly and repeat. Keep going until you have covered your whole head – your fingers will meet in the middle of your scalp. Repeat this process at least twice, and feel the energy tingle under your fingers. (This is also great for a hangover.)

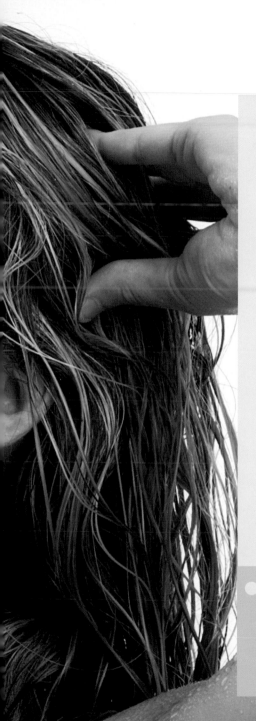

CARDAMOM & GRAPEFRUIT AROMATHERAPY SKIN BLEND

Pour 4 teaspoons grapeseed carrier oil into a small bowl. Add 4 drops cardamom and 6 drops grapefruit essential oils, and stir. This is a non-greasy aromatherapy blend, thanks to the properties of grapeseed, which nourishes the skin without leaving a residue. Cardamom is a beautiful, sweet spice oil that stimulates the circulation, while grapefruit is bright and refreshing, complementing the skin scrub. Apply your blend to dry skin all over your body in soft, circular movements, especially to areas you exfoliated. It leaves the skin silky soft and should not stain your clothes. The delicate fragrance will stay with you through the day.

BANANA & ORANGE SMOOTHIE

Place 1 chopped banana, the grated rind and juice of 1 orange and 6 tablespoons natural yogurt in a blender. Whizz for a few seconds and spoon into a glass. Bananas are rich in B vitamins, as well as potassium, calcium and magnesium – vital minerals for concentration – and oranges contain vitamin C.

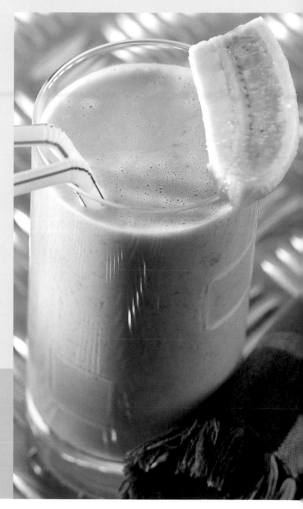

●●● TREATMENT ADVICE

Use home spa treatments on the day of making. Avoid contact with the eyes. If the treatment gets into the eyes, rinse well with warm water.

GIRLIE SPA DAY: SUPER PAMPER TIME

This is a whole-day routine designed so that you and a group of friends can have a fabulous time making up natural treatment recipes and giving each other massages, as well as enjoying delicious, healthy food. This home spa session is ideal for 4 girls working in pairs, but there can be more of you if you have enough space available. Some of the treatments you give and receive in pairs while others you give to yourself.

GIRLIE SPA MENU
Make up the recipes as you go – it's part of the fun!

BREAKFAST: dishes of luscious prepared sliced fruit, for example pineapple, mango, papaya, banana, strawberries, grapes, and kiwi fruit

MORNING TREATMENTS
Foot pre-treatment: Rosemary Herbal Foot Soak and Olive Oil & Lavender Foot Scrub [see pages 32–3]
Foot massage: Lavender & Lemon Aromatherapy Foot Blend [see pages 34–5]
Face mask treatment: Green Clay & Orange Toning Mask or the Oatmeal, Yogurt & Geranium Mask [see pages 36–7]

Facial treat routine: Infused Chamomile Toner and face massage with Geranium & Grapefruit Face Blend [see page 37]

LUNCH: a large mixed salad for everyone with plenty of raw vegetables drizzled with olive oil and lemon juice; eat it with hummus or vegetable pâté and oatcakes or rice cakes

AFTERNOON TREATMENTS
Hand pre-treatment: Sugar & Lemon Exfoliating Scrub or Ylang Ylang Warm Oil Hand Soak [see page 39]
Hand massage: Ylang Ylang & Lavender Hand Massage Blend [see pages 40–1]

GROUP RELAXATION EXERCISE [see pages 42–3]

HEALTHY SNACK SUGGESTION: a mix of dates, dried apricots, raisins and almonds

DRINK SUGGESTIONS: fresh herb teas such as peppermint or melissa; fresh fruit juices such as orange, apple or grapefruit; also drink several glasses of mineral water

INGREDIENTS:

fresh herbs –
    rosemary, melissa,
    peppermint

full cream milk

extra virgin olive oil

fine sea salt

essential oils –
    lavender, lemon,
    geranium, grapefruit
    and ylang ylang

apricot kernel
    carrier oil

green clay powder

organic oranges and
    lemons

fine oatmeal

natural yogurt

chamomile flowers

granulated sugar

fresh fruit

salad ingredients

hummus or vegetable
    pâté

rice or oatcakes

dried fruit

almonds

fruit juices

mineral water

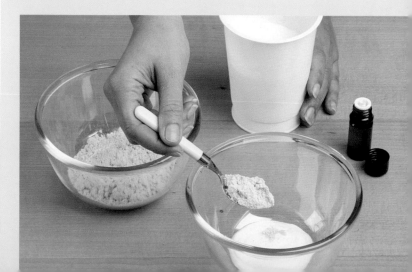

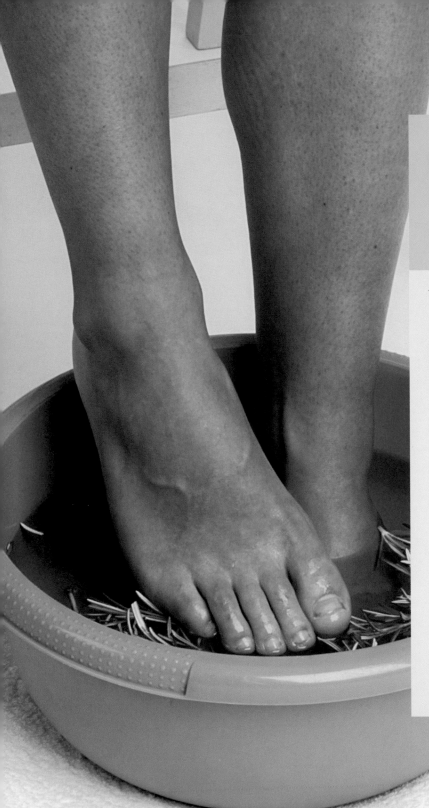

GIRLIE SPA PART 1: FOOT SOAK AND SCRUB

It's good to start your spa day with a foot treatment because it makes you sit down and relax. Dress in a robe or a loose tracksuit so that it's easy for your partner to work with you when it's your turn. For all the foot treatments, your partner needs to sit in a comfortable chair. You will need to have ready a plastic bowl for the foot soak, some towels to dry the feet and some kitchen paper to rest them on while you apply the foot scrub and to wipe away any excess.

● ● ● **TREATMENT ADVICE**
Use home spa treatments on the day of making. Avoid contact with the eyes. If the treatment gets into the eyes, rinse well with warm water.

ROSEMARY HERBAL FOOT SOAK

Pour comfortably warm water into a plastic bowl so that it is half full. Add a handful of washed and chopped fresh rosemary leaves, and place your partner's feet in the bowl. As the leaves infuse into the liquid and bathe the feet, they gently deodorize and tone the skin. Leave the feet to soak for 15 minutes; if your partner has very dry heels, you could rub a pumice stone gently on the hard skin to smooth it. Then lift your partner's feet out on to a towel and dry them thoroughly

As an option, you can add 6 tablespoons full cream milk to the water. This softens the skin and gives a hint of luxury. (Remember, Cleopatra was known to bathe in asses' milk.)

OLIVE OIL & LAVENDER FOOT SCRUB

In a small bowl, pour 6 tablespoons extra virgin olive oil. Add 2 teaspoons fine sea salt – as an exfoliator – and stir. Add 20 drops lavender essential oil, and stir. Rest your partner's feet on kitchen paper on top of a towel. Then carefully apply the scrub to 1 foot at a time, using small circular movements all over the foot, concentrating especially on any dry areas. The olive oil is supremely nourishing, especially to dry skin, and the lavender is also skin replenishing and

soothing. When you have done this for about 10 minutes, use the kitchen paper to wipe off any excess scrub. The feet should already feel much silkier and ready for the foot massage [see page 34].

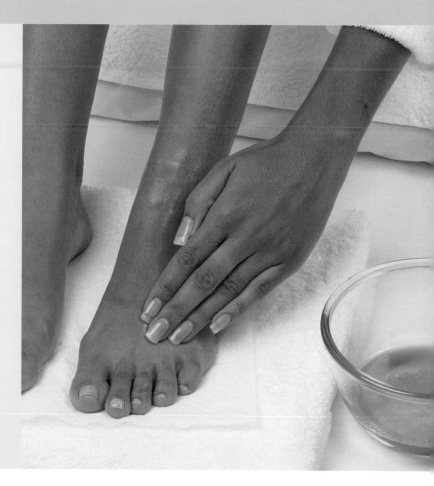

GIRLIE SPA PART 2: FOOT TREAT

Here is a foot massage routine that you can give your partner; it improves circulation, helps stiffness and nourishes the skin. Sit opposite your partner with a towel over your knees, resting her feet on your lap. Massage 1 foot completely first, then the other. Finally, wrap the feet in a towel and let your partner rest.

LEMON AND LAVENDER AROMATHERAPY FOOT BLEND

In a small bowl pour 4 teaspoons apricot kernel carrier oil and add 4 drops lemon and 6 drops lavender essential oils. Stir and use immediately. Apricot kernel is a light, yet rich oil that helps to heal cracked or dry skin; lavender eases aching feet and lemon gently tones.

TREATMENT ADVICE

Use home spa treatments on the day of making. Avoid contact with the eyes. If the treatment gets into the eyes, rinse well with warm water.

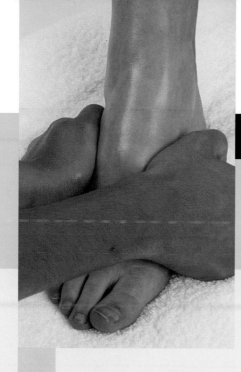

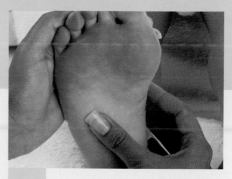

1 Apply at least 1 teaspoon foot blend all over the surface of the foot. Working on the upper side of the foot, use both hands to squeeze the whole area, easing out to the sides, applying firm pressure. Check with your partner that this feels comfortable. This movement eases stiffness and warms the foot.

2 Use your left hand to support the foot underneath. With your right thumb, trace steady lines of pressure from the base of the toes up towards the ankle. This may be a little tender, so be careful; these are drainage strokes, which help the lymphatic vessels in the foot. Do 3 sets of stripes, feeling carefully between the tendons.

3 Working on the lower surface of the foot, use your thumb to make slow circles of pressure over the ball, arch and heel; work from the big toe side out towards the little toe. This pressure eases out the bones in the foot, which may be cramped due to poorly fitting shoes. Firm pressure is not ticklish and should feel comfortable.

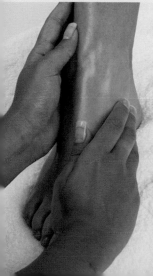

4 Just stroke the foot all over with both hands, really nurturing and nourishing all the surfaces, including the toes. This eases the foot after the first 2 sets of movements. Work the foot blend really well into any dry areas, especially the heels.

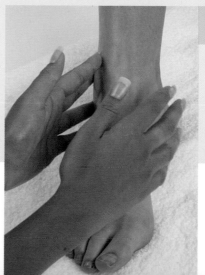

5 Using both hands, tap the foot lightly all over to stimulate the circulation, then stroke it to soothe. Repeat the whole routine on the other foot, then wrap both feet in a towel while your partner rests.

GIRLIE SPA PART 3: FACIAL CARE

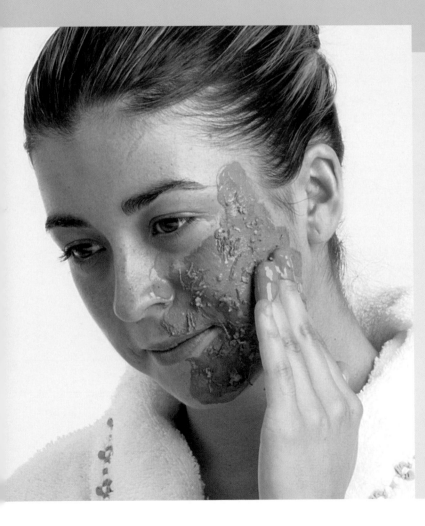

Here is a lovely facial routine – mask, tone and nourish – which you give to yourself. The mask draws out impurities, the toner soothes and hydrates and the final step is an aromatherapy face massage blend. Using natural ingredients on the face is wonderfully refreshing.

A CHOICE OF MASKS

Green Clay & Orange Toning Mask
(for greasy or combination skin)

In a small bowl put 2 teaspoons green clay powder. Add the grated rind and freshly squeezed juice of an orange, and stir to a paste – add a little water if you need more liquid. The green clay is an excellent skin purifier, and the orange gently tones the pores.

Oatmeal, Yogurt & Geranium Mask
(for dry or mature skin)

In a small bowl put 2 teaspoons fine oatmeal, 3 teaspoons natural yogurt and 3 drops geranium essential oil; mix to a paste. Oatmeal is soothing and anti-inflammatory, yogurt is cooling and hydrating and geranium oil balances the skin's natural oils.

MASK APPLICATION

First, moisten the skin with warm water on a cotton wool pad. Then apply the mask all over the face, avoiding the eye area. Leave for 15 minutes, then remove with warm water and pat the skin dry.

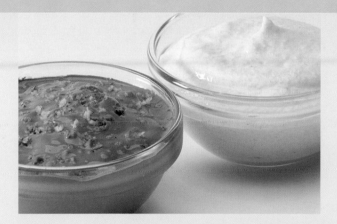

TONE
Infused Chamomile Toner

In a small heatproof dish put 1 teaspoon dried or 2 teaspoons fresh chamomile flowers. Pour 100 ml near-boiling water over them, place a saucer over the liquid and leave for 15 minutes to infuse; strain, then refrigerate. Apply to the skin with cotton wool pads to soothe the skin after the mask.

NOURISH
Geranium & Grapefruit Face Blend

In a small dish pour 4 teaspoons apricot kernel carrier oil; add 2 drops geranium and 4 drops grapefruit essential oils, and stir. Apricot kernel is a lovely light, yet rich, carrier for facial massage; geranium soothes the skin and grapefruit refreshes and tones. This gentle blend can be used on all skin types. This recipe will do 4 face treatments, so make up more blend as necessary. Apply the blend all over your face in tiny circular movements from forehead to chin. After this treatment, lie down and rest for 10 minutes – listen to some soothing music. [Melissa or peppermint herbal teas can also help you to relax.]

●●● TREATMENT ADVICE

Use home spa treatments on the day of making. Avoid contact with the eyes. If the treatment gets into the eyes, rinse well with warm water.

GIRLIE SPA
PART 4: HAND EXFOLIATION OR SOAK

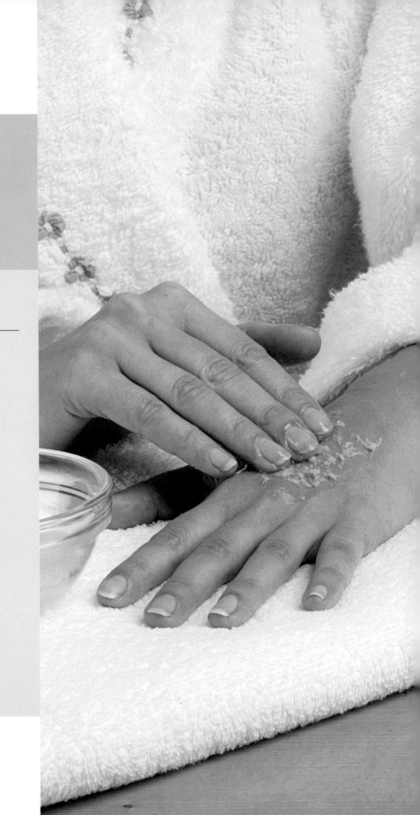

It is surprising how relaxing it is to receive a hand treatment. Hands work very hard performing thousands of repetitive tasks each day; they are also exposed to many types of chemicals in soaps and detergents. The skin on the hands becomes easily dehydrated. Here you have the choice between a gentle exfoliation and a warm oil hand soak to prepare the hands for a massage. For the scrub, let your partner sit in a comfortable chair, resting her hands on a towel; for the soak, she needs to sit at a table.

SUGAR & LEMON EXFOLIATING SCRUB

This is so scrummy that you will have trouble not eating it. In a small glass bowl put 2 tablespoons granulated sugar; add the rind of 1 organic lemon and 1 tablespoon lemon juice, then 2 tablespoons apricot kernel carrier oil. Stir together. Sugar granules gently exfoliate the skin, and lemon juice and rind tone and cleanse; apricot kernel is soothing and nourishing. Apply a small amount and work gently into the hands, including all the fingers. Then wipe off any excess with a damp paper towel. This quantity should be enough to do 2 pairs of hands; make up more as needed.

YLANG YLANG WARM OIL HAND SOAK

Pour enough near-boiling water to half fill a medium-sized heatproof bowl. Then in a smaller heatproof bowl pour 4 teaspoons apricot kernel carrier and add 4 drops ylang ylang essential oil. Stand the small dish in the larger bowl of hot water to warm the oil. Then lift the small dish out of the bowl and soak each hand in the warm oil for around 5 minutes. Wipe off any excess with a damp paper towel. Ylang Ylang is a skin-conditioning essential oil that creates a lovely exotic floral aroma somewhat like jasmine. This quantity of soak will do 2 pairs of hands; you may need to re-warm it for the second person.

●●● TREATMENT ADVICE

Use home spa treatments on the day of making. Avoid contact with the eyes. If the treatment gets into the eyes, rinse well with warm water.

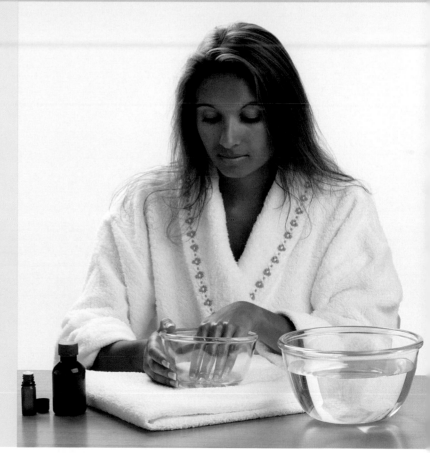

GIRLIE SPA PART 5: HAND MASSAGE

This is a treat, especially after the preparation of the exfoliation or soak. Your partner needs to relax in an armchair, letting her hand rest on a towel. Sit on the same side as the hand you are massaging, so that you can be comfortable. If you have long nails, try to use the pads of your fingers rather than the tips to apply pressure.

Try a Mango & Yogurt Shake in between sessions: in a blender whizz together the flesh of 1 mango with 4 tablespoons natural yogurt and 120 ml/4 fl oz full cream milk...delicious!

YLANG YLANG & LAVENDER HAND MASSAGE BLEND

In a small bowl pour 4 teaspoons apricot kernel oil; add 3 drops ylang ylang and 7 drops lavender essential oils, and stir. In the light, rich, apricot carrier oil, ylang ylang conditions the skin and lavender eases aches and stiffness. This quantity should be enough to massage 4 pairs of hands.

● ● ● TREATMENT ADVICE
Use home spa treatments on the day of making. Avoid contact with the eyes. If the treatment gets into the eyes, rinse well with warm water.

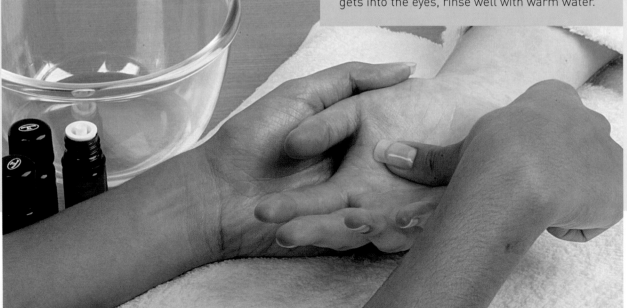

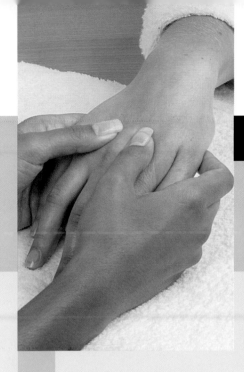

HAND MASSAGE ROUTINE

1 Gently apply half a teaspoon of the blend, stroking it all over the hand. Then use both your hands to squeeze the upper surface of your partner's hand firmly from the middle out to the sides. This eases out the bones and loosens the muscles. Check that the pressure is comfortable.

2 Still on the upper surface of your partner's hand, and supporting it underneath with your fingers, use your thumbs to make lines of steady pressure from the knuckles up towards the wrist. Work from each knuckle in turn, and repeat this sequence twice. These strokes help to encourage lymphatic drainage from the hand.

3 Supporting with 1 hand, use your other hand to squeeze and massage each of your partner's fingers and thumb in turn. Really take time over this, working the blend into the nail area as well as all over the fingers. Apricot kernel carrier is very nourishing to the cuticles and nails.

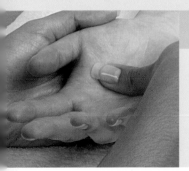

4 Turn your partner's hand over; use your thumb to make slow deep circles all the way around the surface of the palm itself. This area is full of sensitive nerve endings, so this stroke is very soothing to receive. It also eases out tension and stress from the hand.

5 Sandwich your partner's hand between both of yours and stroke both surfaces of the hand together, really warming and soothing the whole area. Ease off gently, wrap the hand in a towel and repeat the routine on the other hand.

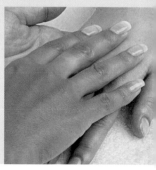

GIRLIE SPA PART 6: RELAXATION EXERCISE

By the end of this one-day session, with hands, feet and faces glowing, you should feel wonderfully pampered and your digestive system should have enjoyed a real treat from the healthy lunch and lush fruit snacks. You will have had fun and laughs using all the natural recipes and you will be feeling the benefits of silkier and smoother skin. Here is a relaxation exercise to do together to round off your home spa day.

RELAXATION EXERCISE

Find a space to lie down on the floor; use a flat cushion or a folded towel to support your head. Wear a loose tracksuit or put a shawl over you to keep warm, as you are going to be lying down for about 20 minutes. You might like to record the meditation so that you can listen to, rather than read, the instructions.

EXERCISE INSTRUCTIONS

1 Lie on your back, with your arms loose and comfortable by your sides. Feel how your body lies on the ground; notice any areas of tension; breathe into them regularly and quietly, imagining you are sending warmth into them, dissolving the tension. Do this for a few moments.

2 Now, beginning at your feet, slowly stretch your toes upwards and circle your feet first one way, then the other. Then let the feet relax.
* Tense your legs for 5 seconds, feeling the pull in every muscle, then relax the legs.
* Clench your buttocks for 5 seconds, tightly, then relax them.
* Stretch out your hands – flex your fingers; now make circles with both hands, first one way, then the other, then relax.
* Tense both your arms, really tight, then let them flop.

* Bring both your shoulders up towards your ears, really squeeze...then relax.
* Gently and slowly move your head from side to side, then relax back to centre.
* Finally, tense up your face for a few seconds, then relax.

3 Breathe gently, and imagine there is a smile inside your head. Feel energy circulating and tingling throughout your body. You have nourished and cared for yourself today, and your whole system has been rejuvenated.

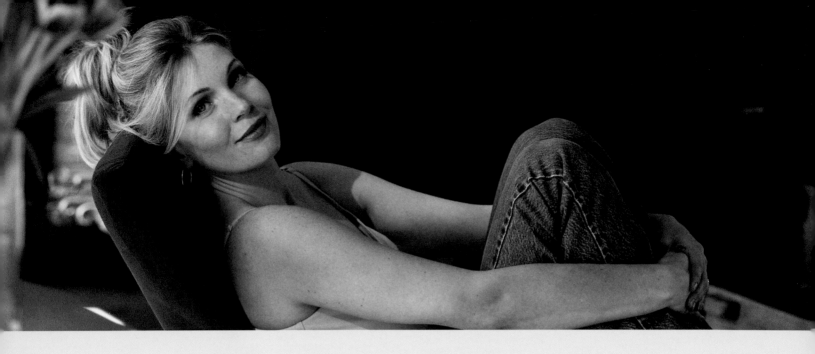

SOLO SPA DAY: RELAX AND RETREAT

Sometimes it's simply wonderful to spend time alone. This allows you to decide what you do and when you do it, following your own internal flow. This is a one-day solo spa routine, which will help you to rediscover your own inner rhythms while you recover from the demands of everyday life. A combination of treatments, dietary suggestions, gentle exercise and relaxation will renew your body and mind. Make sure you will not be disturbed so that you receive the full benefits. The night before you begin, drink 2 or 3 glasses of mineral water an hour before bed, and try to eat lightly.

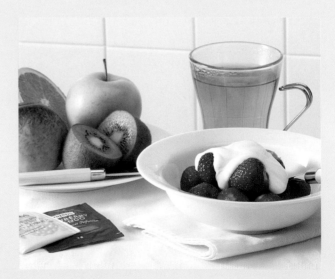

SOLO SPA MENU

Make up the recipes in advance.

FIRST THING IN THE MORNING: a mug of boiling water with a slice of lemon; this starts the cleansing process

BREAKFAST: a choice of seasonal fruit and natural yogurt sprinkled with sunflower seeds; herbal tea, such as chamomile or fennel

MORNING TREATMENTS: a detoxifying Marjoram, Rosemary & Lavender Milk Bath and a self-massage with rich aromatherapy Ylang Ylang, Lemon & Grapefruit Jojoba Body Blend [see page 47]

REST TIME: relaxation with music

LUNCH: a large raw salad with detoxifying green leaves, carrot, celery and radish, dressed with olive oil and lemon juice; choose between hard-boiled egg, hummus or vegetable pâté with your salad; follow with a choice of fresh fruit or Greek yogurt drizzled with honey

EARLY AFTERNOON: a one-hour walk in nature: spend time in your garden, go to a park or walk by the sea

LATE AFTERNOON TREATMENTS: full facial including a Chamomile & Melissa Facial Steam, an Avocado, Cypress & Lavender Nourishing Mask, an Almond, Honey & Lemon Facial Scrub, and a Melissa Herbal Toner [see pages 48–9]; followed by a special face massage routine with Geranium & Jojoba Skin Balm [see pages 50–1]

REST TIME: relaxation before dinner

DINNER: grilled chicken or salmon seasoned with lemon juice and black pepper, with 120 g /4 oz cooked plain rice and a selection of lightly steamed vegetables, such as broccoli, carrots and mangetout; follow with a dish of sliced fresh pineapple

EVENING: meditation exercise [see pages 52–3].

INGREDIENTS

fresh marjoram, chamomile, rosemary and melissa
Dead Sea mineral salts
full cream milk
lavender, ylang ylang, grapefruit, lemon, cypress and geranium essential oils
jojoba carrier oil
avocado
organic lemon
ground almonds
honey
seasonal fruits and salad ingredients
natural yogurt
sunflower seeds
chamomile or fennel herb tea
free-range eggs, hummus or vegetable pâté
chicken or salmon fillet
fresh vegetables
mineral water

SOLO SPA
PART 1:
GENTLE DETOX

After a gentle start to the day and a light breakfast, the first part of your solo pampering time is spent in a wonderful detoxifying bath. A combination of herbs and essential oil in the water, along with milk to soften the skin, creates a gorgeous aroma in your bathroom, and the time you spend in the water helps you to appreciate the slower pace of the day. Have some music playing while you are in the water, and even though it is morning, light a small candle – it makes the space feel very restful and special. After the bath you are going to nourish your skin with a rich aromatherapy blend.

MARJORAM, ROSEMARY & LAVENDER MILK BATH

Wash and trim a generous handful of fresh marjoram and rosemary leaves and chop them up; mix them in a saucer with 2 tablespoons Dead Sea mineral salts (these help the detoxifying process). Run the bath to a comfortable temperature, and add 6 tablespoons full cream milk to the water. Then add the salt and herb mix, and swish it into the water; finally, add 3 drops lavender essential oil before getting in. Marjoram and rosemary have a toning and relaxing effect, complemented by lavender's soothing properties. Soak and relax for at least 20 minutes. Towards the end of the bath, use a good quality soap to lather your skin.

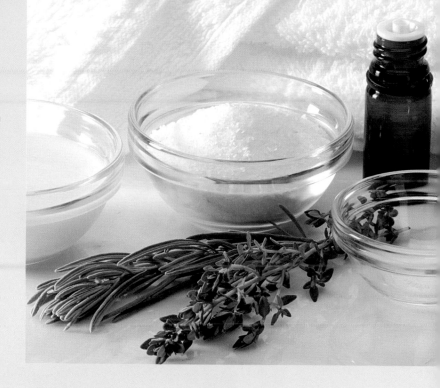

YLANG YLANG, LEMON & GRAPEFRUIT JOJOBA BODY BLEND

Pour 4 teaspoons jojoba carrier oil into a small bowl. Add 3 drops each ylang ylang, grapefruit and lemon essential oils, and stir. This is a delicate citrus and floral blend that has an uplifting effect on the mind, while the jojoba is one of the most wonderful carriers, a liquid wax with extremely beneficial effects on all skin types – even greasy. Its golden colour gives a feeling of luxury. Dry your skin well and sit on a fluffy towel. Then, starting at your feet, apply the blend in smooth, sweeping strokes over your feet, up your legs and arms, and over your whole body. Take time over knees, elbows, heels – anywhere the skin is dry.

When you have finished, wrap up in a soft robe and shawls and rest comfortably, letting all these beneficial ingredients do their work. Drink a large glass of water. Listen to some music that encourages you to relax. Just before lunch, get dressed in loose comfortable clothes.

●○○● TREATMENT ADVICE

Use home spa treatments on the day of making. Avoid contact with the eyes. If the treatment gets into the eyes, rinse well with warm water.

SOLO SPA PART 2: FACIAL PAMPER

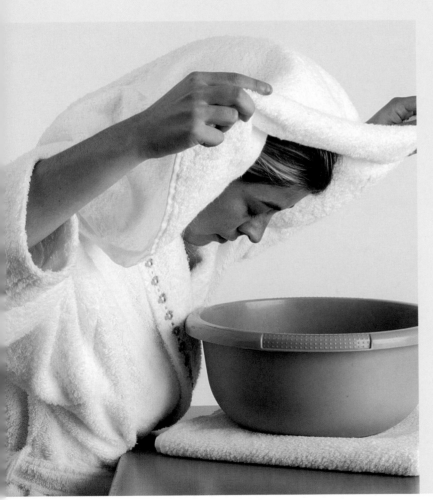

After lunch, you will have spent some time outside in nature; later in the afternoon, you are going to give yourself a fabulous facial. This routine – steam, mask, scrub and tone – is full of simple yet beneficial natural ingredients, which care for all skin types. It prepares the skin for the face massage on pages 50–1.

CHAMOMILE & MELISSA FACIAL STEAM

Wash and chop a handful of fresh melissa leaves and chamomile flowers. Pour near-boiling water into a medium-sized heatproof bowl until it is half full. Scatter the herbs on the surface of the water, then lean over the bowl with your face in the steam and your head under a towel. Steam opens up your pores and eliminates impurities, while melissa and chamomile are extremely soothing to the skin. Stay under the towel for about 15 minutes, then wipe your face with a damp flannel and pat it dry.

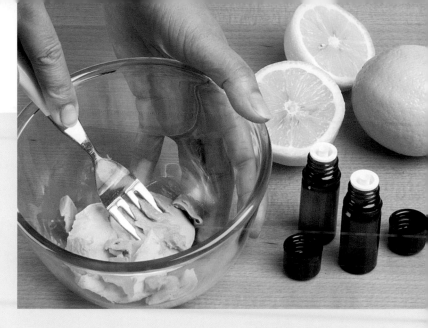

AVOCADO, CYPRESS & LAVENDER NOURISHING MASK

In a small bowl mash up the flesh of half a ripe avocado, add 1 teaspoon lemon juice, then 2 drops cypress and 3 drops lavender essential oils. Avocado is full of vitamins A, D and E, which nourish and protect the skin. Lemon juice and cypress tone the pores, and lavender soothes the skin. Apply the rich green paste all over the face, avoiding the eye area. Leave on for 15 minutes, then wash off with tepid water and pat the skin dry.

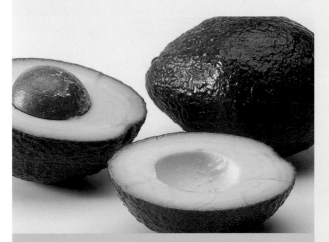

● ● ● TREATMENT ADVICE

Use home spa treatments on the day of making. Avoid contact with the eyes. If the treatment gets into the eyes, rinse well with warm water.

ALMOND, HONEY & LEMON FACIAL SCRUB

To make this gentle exfoliator, [in a saucer] put 2 tablespoons ground almonds (if you are allergic to nuts, substitute fine oatmeal), 2 tablespoons good quality honey and 2 tablespoons lemon juice. Mix together, then apply to the face in small circular movements, avoiding the eye area. Ground almonds remove dead cells and smooth the skin; honey is hydrating and lemon juice tones the pores. Leave on for 15 minutes, then wash off with warm water.

MELISSA HERBAL TONER

Prepare a melissa infusion by putting 2 tablespoons chopped fresh leaves in a small heatproof bowl. Pour over 180 ml/6 fl oz boiling water, allow to infuse for 15 minutes, strain, then refrigerate. Apply the infusion to the skin with a cotton wool pad and feel the freshening effect of the melissa.

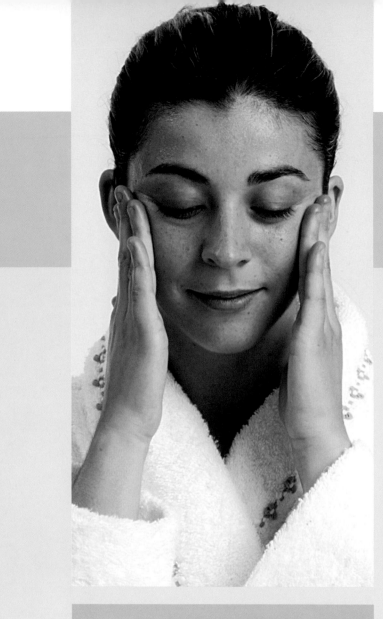

SOLO SPA PART 3: FACIAL MASSAGE

This is a luxurious face massage, which nourishes your skin as well as working on underlying facial muscles to tone and uplift. The blend uses jojoba as a carrier – a rich, golden, liquid skin food. You should find that your skin is soft and moist after the previous preparation and ready to receive the deep nourishment of the massage. Make sure your hair is tied back off your forehead before you start the routine.

An even more luxurious version of this massage can be done with pure rose essential oil – 2 drops in 2 teaspoons jojoba carrier.

GERANIUM & JOJOBA SKIN BALM

Pour 4 teaspoons jojoba carrier oil into a small dish. Add 4 drops geranium essential oil, and stir. Geranium balances and hydrates all skin types. You can also use this blend for night-time skin massages after the end of your home spa.

● ● ○ TREATMENT ADVICE

Use home spa treatments on the day of making. Avoid contact with the eyes. If the treatment gets into the eyes, rinse well with warm water.

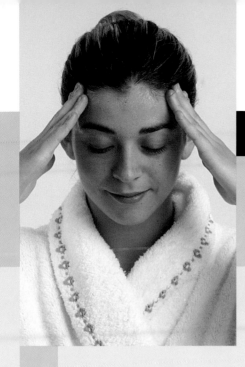

FACE MASSAGE ROUTINE

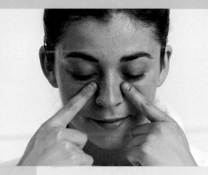

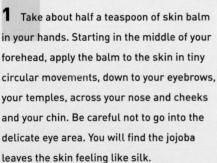

1 Take about half a teaspoon of skin balm in your hands. Starting in the middle of your forehead, apply the balm to the skin in tiny circular movements, down to your eyebrows, your temples, across your nose and cheeks and your chin. Be careful not to go into the delicate eye area. You will find the jojoba leaves the skin feeling like silk.

2 Using your index fingers only, start in the middle of your eyebrows and apply gentle pressure in a circle all around the bony eye socket area; this area contains many acupressure points that link to the lungs and the digestive system. This sequence helps elimination.

3 Continue applying gentle pressure down the sides of your nose, across your cheeks, around your mouth, down to your chin and along your jaw. This pressure also stimulates fresh blood supply to your skin. Your face should feel quite tingly.

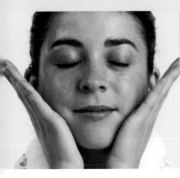

4 Using the palms of your hands, sweep up the neck towards the chin in light, alternating, feathery movements. Use your fingertips to tap lightly all over your face, which gently stimulates the skin.

5 Gently stroke all over the face in soft circular movements to finish, feeling the softness of your skin. This kind of deep nourishment is vital for repair and renewal, whatever your skin type. The jojoba should leave no tackiness, just a smooth, even skin surface.

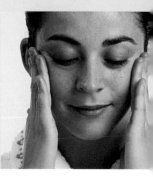

SOLO SPA: MEDITATION EXERCISE

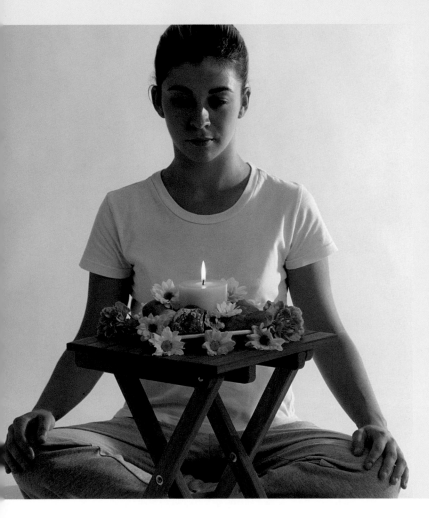

After dinner, and at the end of a day of relaxing and nurturing treatment, it is good to prepare for bed with a simple but very effective meditation exercise. The aim of the solo home spa has been to completely unwind your body and your mind, and you should feel very rested. Mental relaxation is as important as physical; the brain controls the chemical balance of the body, and in a relaxed state the balance changes from hyperactivity to calmness. This, in turn, benefits the heart and the whole nervous system. Meditation is simply contemplation; if you have never tried it, have a go. The simple focus it brings will surprise you.

To get ready, wear warm, loose clothing, and perhaps a shawl around your shoulders. If you are comfortable sitting cross-legged on the floor, then adopt this pose; otherwise, sit on a hard-backed dining chair with both feet on the ground and your hands resting gently in your lap. On a table in front of you, place a candle in the middle of a dinner plate. Add a few beach pebbles or fresh flowers to create a simple display. Dim the lights and light the candle.

Sit comfortably and focus your gaze on the candle display. Let the soft light bathe your eyes, and look right into the flame. Candlelight is soothing to the eyes, yet in the very middle of the flame it is extremely bright; at the edges you may even see traces of blue. Each time your concentration wanders, bring it back to the flame. Be gentle with yourself the first time you do this exercise; just keep your eyes on the centre. You may begin to feel very relaxed, and conscious of your breathing or your heartbeat – this is normal, just allow it. Sit for about 15 minutes, then stretch your fingers and toes and bring your awareness back into the present.

MEDITATE REGULARLY

Regular meditation is very helpful both early in the morning and late at night. Getting into a pattern of this kind will help you to cope much more effectively with stress.

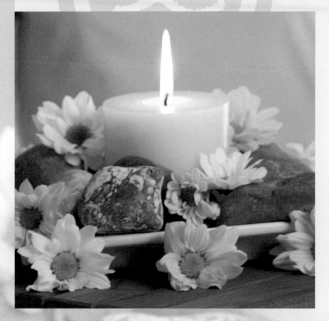

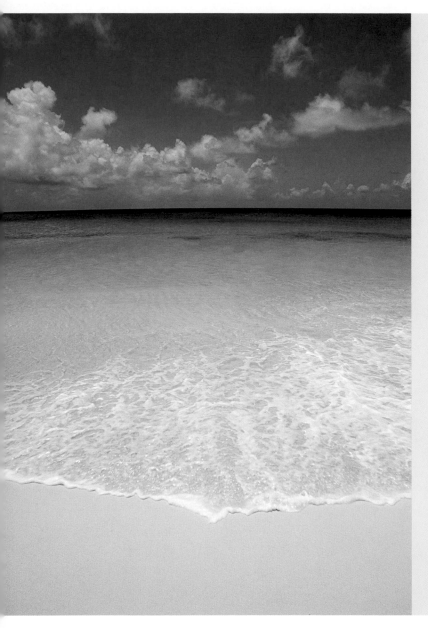

TWO-HOUR EVENING SPA: REFRESH BODY AND MIND

Here is a home spa routine that really transforms an evening into some special nurturing time. Instead of collapsing in front of the television at the end of the day, in just 2 hours you can feel transformed. Start your evening with a light but tasty dinner; this is a tonic for your taste buds and improves your mood. Then a hair wrap is a luxurious treat, especially when essential oils are also used to condition the scalp. The hair is wonderfully perfumed and soft afterwards. A toning shower with uplifting essential oils is a great way to refresh both body and mind, followed by a neck and shoulder massage to ease out daily tension, neck pain and stiffness. The evening ends with a lovely visualization exercise to help you unwind mentally; creative visualization is a wonderful technique for refreshing your thinking.

TWO-HOUR EVENING SPA MENU

Although this session is presented as a solo session, there is no reason why you could not share it with a friend or partner. You could also think about repeating it once a week as a special treat, particularly if you are having a pressurized time at work. It is amazing how a short session like this can make all the difference to your mood, your sleep and your concentration the following day. You could vary the dinner menu and alternate the shower treatment with the Marjoram, Rosemary & Lavender Milk Bath on page 47.

Make up the recipes in advance.

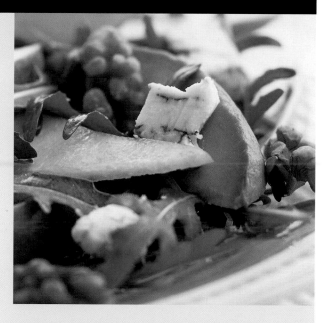

DINNER: prepare a nutritious mixed salad with avocado or smoked salmon dressed with olive oil and lemon juice; for dessert, blend the flesh of 1 papaya with 120 g/4 oz raspberries, stir in 1 teaspoon honey and 4 tablespoons natural yogurt to make a Papaya & Raspberry Whirl: drink mineral water to accompany the meal and during the session.

TREATMENTS: a Cardamom Hot Oil Hair Wrap; a Juniper & Grapefruit Toning Shower; and a self-given neck and shoulder massage with Lavender & Ylang Ylang Aromatherapy Massage Blend

VISUALIZATION EXERCISE: beach and sea

INGREDIENTS

jojoba and sweet	avocado or smoked
almond carrier oils	salmon
cardamom, juniper,	olive oil
grapefruit,	1 lemon
lavender and ylang	1 papaya
ylang essential oils	raspberries
unperfumed plant-	honey
based shower gel	natural yogurt
salad ingredients	mineral water

TWO-HOUR EVENING SPA PART 1: HAIR AND BODY TREATMENT

Here you will give yourself a hot oil hair treatment, sit and relax with some music, then shower it off. Hot oil treatment is extremely good for the health of the scalp: the heat opens the pores, enabling the carrier to nourish dry areas and the essential oil – in this case cardamon – to stimulate the blood flow to the hair roots, so the hair grows healthy and strong. It is also a very pleasant and relaxing treatment. Follow the instructions carefully and you will end up with wonderful silky, fragrant hair. The second part of the treatment is a Juniper & Grapefruit Toning Shower Gel; make this up before you start so that you can use it straight away.

CARDAMOM HOT OIL HAIR TREATMENT

You work the treatment into DRY hair. Pour enough boiling water into a medium-sized heatproof bowl to half fill it. Into a smaller heatproof dish pour 2 tablespoons jojoba carrier oil; add 6 drops cardamom essential oil, and stir in. Place the small dish in the medium one, resting it in the boiling water to warm the oil. Leave for 5–10 minutes, then scoop the warm fragrant oil into your hands and work it into your dry hair and scalp. When your whole head is covered, take a large piece of cling film and wrap your hair up in it like a turban. Wrap a towel around your head to finish, then sit comfortably and relax for 15 minutes, listening to some music. Your scalp will start to tingle and feel very warm. Unwrap your head carefully, take some good quality shampoo and WORK IT STRAIGHT INTO YOUR HAIR. Don't put water on before or with the shampoo, otherwise it will be very hard to get the oil out. When you have worked up a rich lather, get in the shower and rinse it all away. When you dry your hair, it will smell very fragrant.

JUNIPER & GRAPEFRUIT TONING SHOWER GEL

In a small bowl put 2 tablespoons unperfumed shower gel; add 3 drops juniper and 6 drops grapefruit essential oils, then stir together well. Juniper tones and purifies the skin, and grapefruit is cleansing and refreshing. This shower gel can be applied with a massage glove or a cellulite massager to really work it into problem areas like the hips and thighs. The bright tingling fragrance greatly uplifts the spirits. Use on the day of making. Avoid contact with the eyes. If the product gets into the eyes, rinse well with warm water.

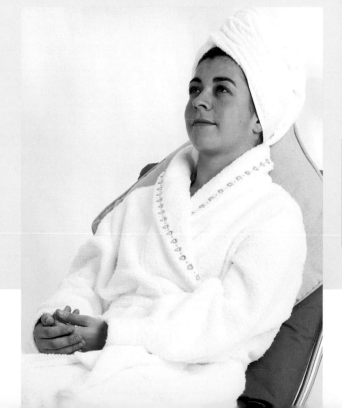

● ● ● ● TREATMENT ADVICE

Use home spa treatments on the day of making. Avoid contact with the eyes. If the treatment gets into the eyes, rinse well with warm water.

TWO-HOUR EVENING SPA
PART 2: NECK AND SHOULDER MASSAGE

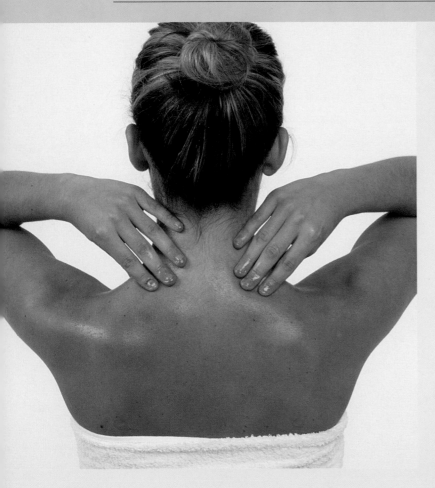

Here you wind down with a lovely simple neck and shoulder massage. To give this routine to yourself, put a towel over the back of a comfortable armchair and sit back so that you can reach your shoulders and spine more easily. You can also do this routine lying down on your bed on a towel.

Remember to drink at least 3 large glasses of water during your evening spa.

LAVENDER & YLANG YLANG AROMATHERAPY MASSAGE BLEND

Pour 4 teaspoons sweet almond carrier oil into a small bowl; add 3 drops lavender and 2 drops ylang ylang essential oils. Stir in, and the blend is ready.

TREATMENT ADVICE

Use home spa treatments on the day of making. Avoid contact with the eyes. If the treatment gets into the eyes, rinse well with warm water.

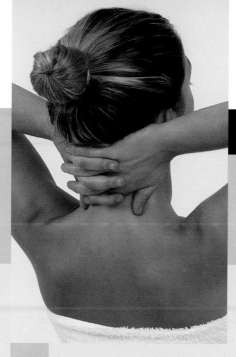

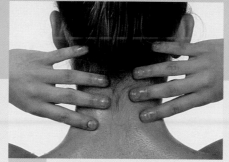

1 Lace your hands behind your neck and lean back to stretch your head and neck gently – don't force it. Then take half a teaspoon of massage blend into your hands and apply it all over your neck and shoulder area to lubricate the skin.

2 Place your fingers on either side of the bones in your neck. These cervical vertebrae carry the weight of your head; assisted by complex groups of muscles, they enable all the movements you make. Now use your fingertips to massage up and down on either side of the bones; you will feel tension easing as you work the area using tiny, precise movements. This step can help to ease headaches.

3 Try to sit so that you are well supported by the chair and your arms are relaxed. Use your fingers to knead across your shoulders; this movement can be quite deep. Your fingers will be doing the work; squeeze the muscles on either side, imagining that they are pliable like dough. Work from the neck out to the sides of the shoulders and back to the middle again, several times.

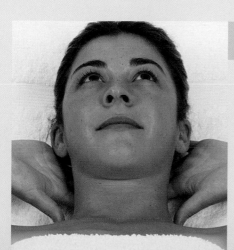

4 Now use your fingers to work as far down as you can, applying pressure in circles to work across the top of the shoulder blades and on either side of the spine. Don't force

the movement: go only as far as you can; if it's too hard to do, go back and do some more shoulder kneading. Finish with some sweeping strokes over the whole area.

TWO-HOUR EVENING SPA
PART 3: VISUALIZATION EXERCISE

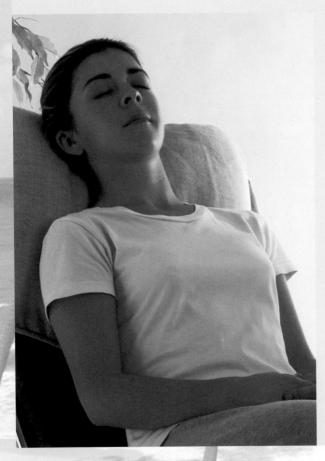

To end your two-hour wind-down session, there is a visualization exercise, which you might like to record so that you can listen to rather than read the instructions. This technique is excellent for calming the mind; it also focuses your attention and stimulates your creative energies. As an aid to the exercise, try vaporizing a combination of essential oils in a diffuser: 2 drops each of lemon, juniper and cardamom is very uplifting. These aromas have a positive effect on mood and help to improve concentration.

Sit comfortably in an armchair, resting your hands on your lap and your head on a cushion. Dim the lights and relax.

BEACH AND SEA VISUALIZATION EXERCISE
Imagine that you are walking on a long stretch of white sandy beach which you can see curving away towards the distant horizon. The temperature is warm and there is a gentle sea breeze. The sun is shining

brightly and you feel very comfortable. You walk slowly, and first you become aware of the sand beneath your toes. It is warm and silky soft to the touch, and every step you take is like a caress. Tiny grains glisten on your skin as you walk along.

You turn to look at the sea. It is quite calm and a deep aquamarine blue, shining with lighter flecks of sunlight. You gaze for a few moments at the stunning blue colour, feeling it bathe your eyes. Then you walk down to the water, smelling the tang of salt, hearing the cry of seabirds and the sound of the waves. Pause for a few moments and let the scene build in your imagination; let your senses create the impressions.

Now imagine that you are going into the water, tasting the salt on your tongue and feeling the tingling, rejuvenating effect of the sea, swimming without effort, still aware of the amazing aquamarine blue colour all around you. Feel how different it is to be in it as well as seeing it. Feel yourself supported by the waves, the sun still shining brightly all around you.

Now come back to the shore and, as you leave the water, feel how refreshed and revitalized you are. Take a few slow, deep breaths, flex your toes and fingers and let your awareness come back to the room.

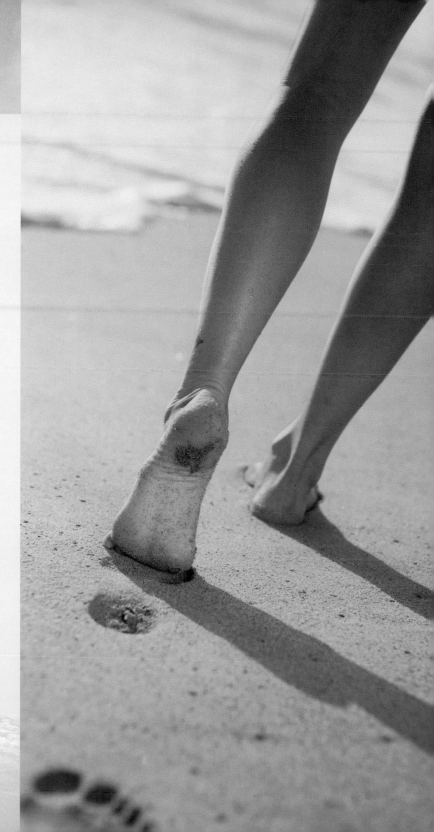

CHAPTER THREE

WEEKEND SPA RETREAT: YOUR OWN OASIS

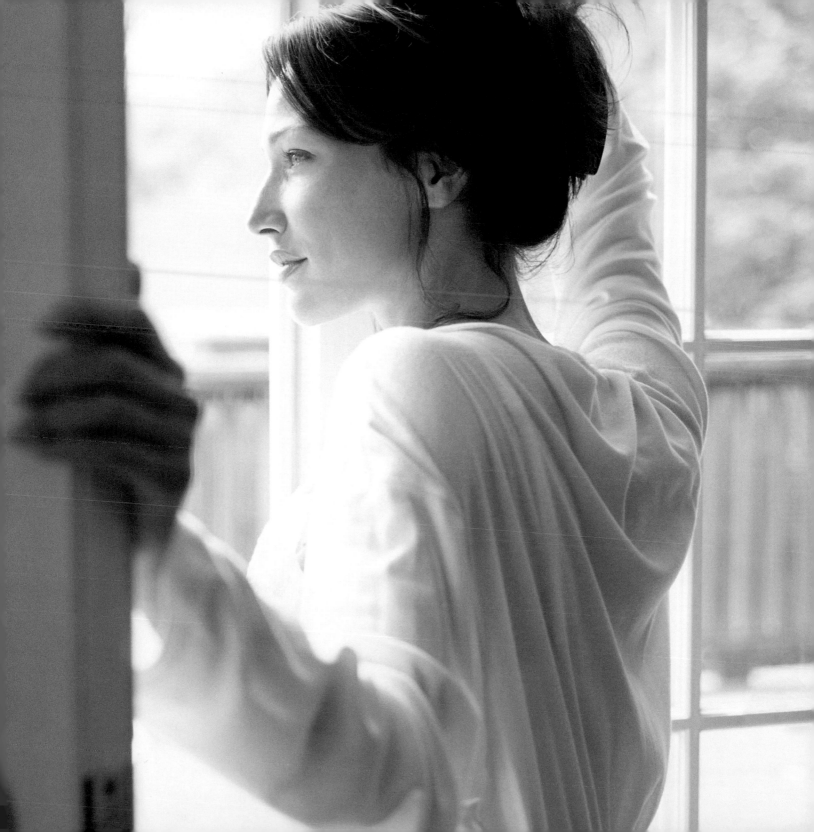

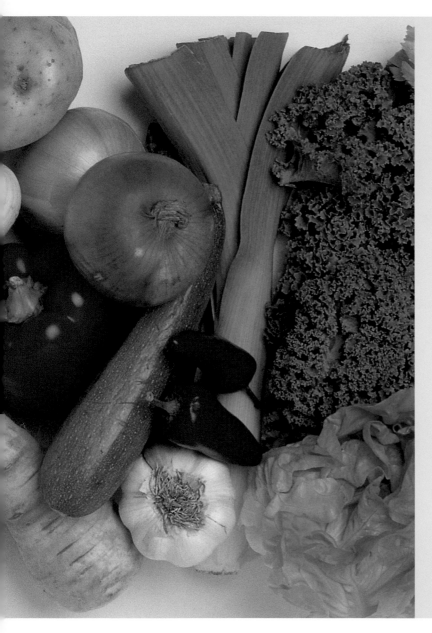

CREATE YOUR WEEKEND SPA RETREAT

H ere is a complete weekend retreat for you to enjoy without having to go to a spa. This takes the concept of home spa to a deeper level; having more time brings you even closer to the spa ideal of balancing inner and outer cleansing treatments. You can use the time to give yourself more in-depth treatments, relax and have periods of activity as well. This two-day programme is designed to concentrate on invigorating treatments in the mornings and relaxing sessions in the afternoons. It works for 2 people, who will give the body treatments to each other.

If you have a recognized medical condition, consult your doctor before attempting this programme.

Here are some things to think about when you plan the time.

NO DISTRACTIONS

This keeps coming up, but it is important. You need to be able to have complete freedom from everyday routine concerns. One way to do this is to organize the home spa weekend for 2 days during a holiday period, when the pressure is off. If you concentrate on the fact that this is a health-giving time for you and your spa partner, then it becomes more than simple pampering: it becomes something you deserve.

EXERCISE

During the two-day programme, there are periods of time designated for exercise. This can be walking in the fresh air, cycling, jogging, swimming or a gym routine, if that is a regular activity for you. The main thing is to choose a form of exercise that you enjoy and feel comfortable doing. In a spa setting, it would be recommended to exercise outdoors as much as possible. Exercise pace should be moderate while on the programme.

DIET

The meals during the 2 days are designed to be light and easily digested, with a cleansing effect. You will find an all-fruit breakfast, a carbohydrate-based lunch and a protein-based evening meal;

spreading key nutrients during the programme like this helps to detoxify the system. Carbohydrate and protein portions should be modest, supplemented by salads, or steamed or stir-fried vegetables. Such simple food takes very little preparation. Use olive oil and lemon juice to dress salads, and a little salt, butter and black pepper to dress steamed vegetables. As ever, drink plenty of mineral water – at least 8 glasses per day.

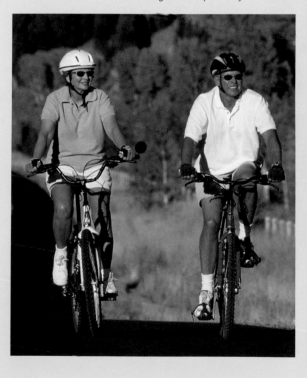

WEEKEND SPA DAY 1
MENU & PART 1: CHINESE EXERCISES

When you are organizing your weekend, you will also need to look at the ingredients needed for Day 2. These can be found on page 76. The night before you begin the retreat, have a light dinner and a relaxing bath or shower, and try to go to bed early. Part 1 starts with some Chinese morning exercises – simple postures to wake up the body's energy.

DAY 1 MENU
Make up the recipes in advance.

ON WAKING: Chinese morning exercises – outside, if possible, for 15 minutes [see opposite]

TREATMENTS
Hot and cold hydrotherapy shower using Peppermint & Rosemary Nourishing Body Scrub [see page 69]

BREAKFAST: a dish of sliced fruit – pineapple, mango, papaya; chamomile herb tea

MORNING EXERCISE: chosen activity for 1 hour; exercise moderately; shower afterwards

MORNING TREATMENT: foot and leg massage using Cypress, Lemon & Juniper Aromatherapy Blend, exchanged between partners [see pages 70–1]

LUNCH: 120 g/4 oz cooked rice per person and stir-fried vegetables with soy sauce, lemon juice and fresh ginger; fresh fruit and natural yogurt

AFTERNOON SIESTA: rest time with music or light reading for 1 hour

AFTERNOON TREATMENTS:
Hot Oil Peppermint Foot Soak
Acupressure-style foot massage, exchanged between partners [40 minutes each] [see pages 72–3]

DINNER: grilled chicken, fish or nut roast with a variety of steamed vegetables; sliced banana, strawberries and natural yogurt drizzled with honey; drink mineral water with meals and throughout the day

AFTER DINNER: colour meditation

SIMPLE CHINESE MORNING EXERCISES

EXERCISE 1: ENERGIZE THE CIRCULATION

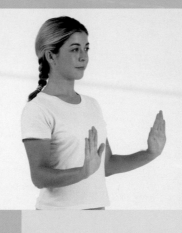

1 Stand relaxed, with elbows bent in by your sides and palms facing out. Breathe easily and naturally.

2 On the out breath, push 1 palm forwards slowly, away from the body, as if resisting pressure. Breathe in and bring the arm back. Repeat with the other arm. Do this on both sides 6 times.

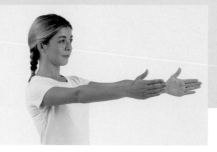

EXERCISE 2: OPEN THE LUNGS

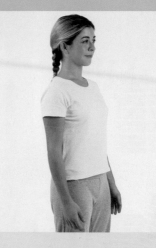

1 Stand relaxed, breathing easily.

2 Point your fingers down to the ground, then raise your arms together slowly, up and over in a circle behind you. Breathe in as you raise your arms and out as you lower them. Repeat 6 times.

INGREDIENTS

unperfumed
   shower gel
fresh herbs –
   peppermint,
   rosemary and
   chamomile
fine sea salt
extra virgin
   olive oil
sweet almond oil
cypress, lemon
   and juniper
   essential oils

fresh fruits
rice
fresh vegetables
soy sauce
lemon juice
fresh ginger
natural yogurt
chicken, fish or
   nut roast
honey

TREATMENT ADVICE

Use home spa treatments on the day of making. Avoid contact with the eyes. If the treatment gets into the eyes, rinse well with warm water.

WEEKEND SPA DAY 1 PART 2: HYDROTHERAPY AND BODY SCRUB

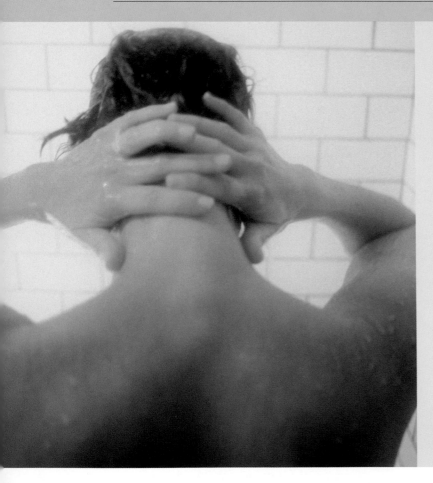

After the simple energy exercises, it is wonderful to start your weekend home spa with a hydrotherapy-style shower session to wake up your whole system. Hydrotherapy techniques have been practised in spas since Greek and Roman times, when warm baths were alternated with ice-cold plunge pools to stimulate and tone the body. In the sauna tradition, the same principle applies: high temperatures encourage detoxification, while exposure to cold water, and even snow, has a really stimulating effect, improving the circulation. The home spa treatment relies on changing the temperature of the shower from warm to cool, which stimulates the circulation under the skin and makes the skin glow. This effect is enhanced by using a special herb body scrub to exfoliate, especially over problem areas, leaving you energized and invigorated. All this before breakfast gives your body a wake-up treat.

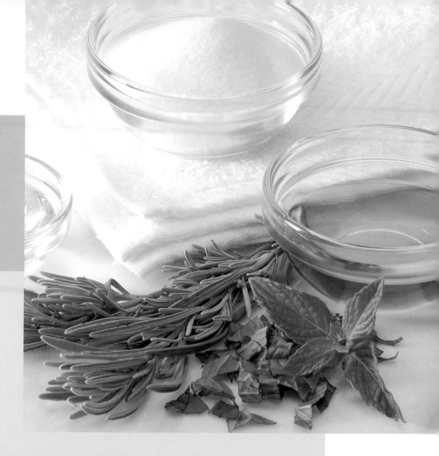

Note: If you have broken or varicose veins, be careful not to pummel them vigorously. Instead, direct the shower jets above or around the area. Also make sure you keep the difference in water temperature moderate – varying only from warm to cool.

PEPPERMINT & ROSEMARY NOURISHING BODY SCRUB

For 2 people, you need 4 tablespoons unperfumed shower gel. Pour this into a small dish and add 2 tablespoons very finely chopped peppermint and rosemary leaves, 1 tablespoon fine sea salt and 1 tablespoon extra virgin olive oil. Stir these ingredients together well. The unperfumed shower gel gives a lathering base; peppermint and rosemary are cleansing and refreshing herbs; sea salt provides the exfoliation and the olive oil adds a skin-nourishing touch to the body scrub.

HOT AND COLD HYDROTHERAPY METHOD

First get in the shower and let the water run comfortably warm; use a little of the herb body scrub to lather up on the skin. Then change the temperature of the water to run much cooler, letting the jets pummel your body, particularly your chest, stomach, buttocks and thighs. This is particularly effective if you have a power shower. Change the temperature back to warm again, and this time apply more of the body scrub, using a cellulite massager to really work it into the skin. Finally, rinse off all the scrub, and towel yourself dry. You should feel very invigorated and refreshed, with soft, glowing skin.

●●● TREATMENT ADVICE

Use home spa treatments on the day of making. Avoid contact with the eyes. If the treatment gets into the eyes, rinse well with warm water.

WEEKEND SPA DAY 1
PART 3: FOOT AND LEG MASSAGE

After your chosen exercise period and shower, it is very refreshing to receive a massage to the legs and feet. This is a very good time for a massage, because the muscles have been well warmed up and the circulation has increased; massage helps to minimize stiffness after exertion, encouraging toxins out of the muscles. The stimulating aromatherapy blend encourages detoxification.

CYPRESS, LEMON & JUNIPER AROMATHERAPY BLEND

Pour 4 teaspoons sweet almond oil into a small dish. Add 3 drops cypress, 4 drops lemon and 3 drops juniper essential oils, and stir in. This will be enough blend to do 2 pairs of legs. Cypress tones the circulation; lemon and juniper encourage elimination.

FOOT AND LEG ROUTINE

Set up the massage with your partner lying face down on the floor on a comfortable mat or futon covered with towels. Rest her head on a pillow. Keep the upper part of the body covered and warm while you work on the legs. Kneel by your partner's feet or by the calves on whichever side feels comfortable to you.

●●● TREATMENT ADVICE
Use home spa treatments on the day of making. Avoid contact with the eyes. If the treatment gets into the eyes, rinse well with warm water.

FOOT AND LEG ROUTINE

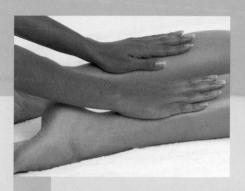

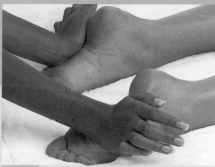

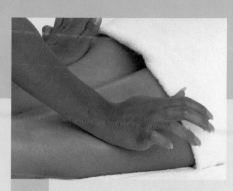

1 Stroke 1 teaspoon of the blend up both legs at the same time, starting from the feet and passing over the ankles, up the calves and thighs, to just below the buttocks. Spread the oil well, and repeat these strokes several times; apply more pressure up the leg and ease off as you come down.

2 Use the heels of your hands to apply slow, firm, circular pressure all over the soles of the feet and then over the calves. This soothing movement works all the main muscle groups.

3 Continue up the legs, using the heels of your hands to apply slow, firm pressure over the backs of the thighs. Be sensitive to your partner and check that the massage is comfortable for her.

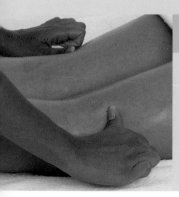

4 Starting above the knees, make vertical lines of individual thumb pressure up towards the buttocks; press for a few moments, then move up a few centimetres and press again. Begin on the outsides of the thighs and work inwards.

5 Repeat the strokes in step 1, using long sweeps up the backs of both legs, with more pressure going up than coming down. Slow down the strokes and ease off to finish.

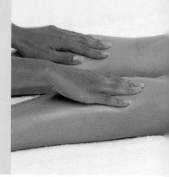

WEEKEND SPA DAY 1
PART 4: FOOT SOAK AND ACUPRESSURE

A really deep foot treatment can be very relaxing indeed. All over the skin surface there are acupressure points that link to the whole body; this is why it makes you feel so good. If you have long nails, be careful to use the pads of your fingers and not the tips. First you give the feet a deep exfoliation, then you follow this with the massage.

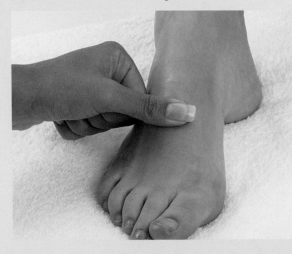

HOT OIL PEPPERMINT FOOT SOAK

You need a plastic bowl large enough to sit both feet in comfortably. You also need a clean jam jar with a screw-top lid. First, wash and very finely chop a handful of fresh peppermint leaves. Put these in the jar, pour over 240 ml/8 fl oz extra virgin olive oil, screw on the lid and shake. Place the jar in a heatproof glass bowl half-filled with boiling water and leave for at least 15 minutes to warm the oil.

Place your partner's feet in the plastic bowl, sprinkle over 2 tablespoons fine sea salt and pour over the warm peppermint-scented oil. While your partner's feet are soaking, rub the salt grains into the skin, covering the whole surface of the feet. The warm olive oil penetrates any cracked skin, while the peppermint is refreshing. After 15 minutes, lift the feet out and wipe them with lots of kitchen roll before wrapping them in a towel. Then move on to the acupressure massage.

ACUPRESSURE-STYLE FOOT MASSAGE

The feet are already lubricated by the soak, so there is no need for more oil. You both need to sit comfortably, your partner's feet should be resting in your lap. Unwrap and work on 1 foot at a time.

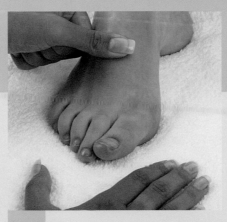

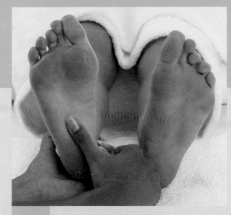

1 Upper foot surface: using your thumbs, apply 5 lines of individual circular pressure from the base of each toe up towards the ankle. Each individual pressure should be firm for a few seconds, then move up slightly and repeat.

2 Lower foot surface: repeat the circular pressure, starting at the base of each toe and pressing down the foot towards the heel. Check with your partner that the treatment feels comfortable – firm, not ticklish.

3 Stroke the foot all over to finish, working over all the surfaces, including the toes. Repeat on the other foot.

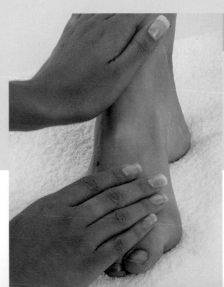

WEEKEND SPA DAY 1
PART 5: COLOUR VISUALIZATION

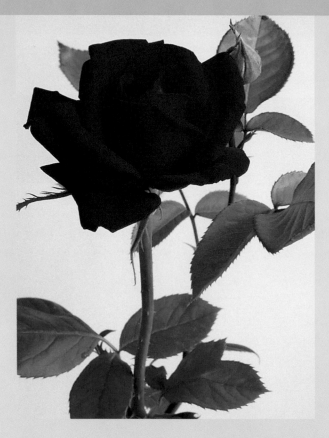

To end your first home spa day, here is a colour visualization that you can use after dinner during a quiet time before bed. You might like to record the visualization so that you can listen to rather than read the instructions. During a spa, watching television is not advised; music or reading or visualization are gentler and more relaxing activities, so do try these for a change. Working with colour is gently soothing in the evening as you unwind. Sit comfortably, and make sure you are warm. Relax, breathing evenly.

COLOUR VISUALIZATION

To begin, enjoy a few quiet moments; release all tension from your thoughts.

First, imagine a rose with deep red petals, velvety and sweetly scented. Concentrate on the rich hues of red, the warmth of the colour, and feel the energy of red enter your body. Notice where you feel it: perhaps you sense a tingling warmth. Pause for a few moments, continuing to visualize the deep red rose.

Next, you see a bright orange marigold, a round-faced daisy with amazing bright petals. The quality of orange is bright, fresh and inviting; let your mind be bathed in the vibrant shades of the marigold flower for just a few moments.

Then you see a buttercup and marvel at its bright golden yellow petals and the golden middle of the flower. Feel the energy of the colour yellow, and how bright and clear it is; notice where you feel it in your body for a few moments.

Now see a patch of velvety green grass, a bright emerald shade. The colour green is very restful to the eyes; feel it bathe your vision. The energy of green is cooling and calming; rest in it for a few moments.

Next, you see a wood full of bluebells, and the blue shade is very soothing and restful to your eyes. Blue is a colour that always has a cooling and calming effect. Pay attention to the amazing blue of the patches of flowers, and feel how you respond to the colour.

Finally, feast your eyes on a field of purple lavender flowers, violet as far as you can see into the horizon, and notice the sensations the colour brings to your vision and to your body. Violet is a tranquil and soft colour, and very easy on the eyes. Notice how your body feels as you visualize violet for a few moments.

Lastly, stretch out your fingers and toes, and slowly bring yourself back to awareness of your surroundings.

WEEKEND SPA DAY 2
MENU AND PART 1: YOGA STRETCHES

Here is the Day 2 menu, which involves a skin detoxifying pack and a deep back massage. Again, the morning is the energizing part of the day, with relaxation time later.

DAY 2 MENU
Make up the recipes in advance.

ON WAKING: morning yoga stretches for 15 minutes [see opposite]

BREAKFAST: fresh sliced strawberries, kiwi fruit, oranges and mango slices; chamomile or peppermint tea

MORNING EXERCISE: moderate exercise as you choose for 1 hour; shower afterwards

MORNING TREATMENTS: detoxifying Thyme, Sage & Juniper Body Mask, applied to each other [see pages 78–9] followed by a massage with Cardamom, Juniper & Lemon Back Massage Blend, given to each other [see pages 80–1]

LUNCH: large mixed salad including cucumber, tomato and watercress; rice or oatcakes and hummus, cottage cheese or hard-boiled egg; banana and natural yogurt sprinkled with sunflower seeds

AFTERNOON SIESTA: 1 hour of relaxation

AFTERNOON EXERCISE: energy postures for the back and neck [see pages 82–3]

DINNER: grilled chicken, fish or nut roast with steamed vegetables; fresh fruit such as pineapple or papaya

EVENING: meditation exercise [see pages 84-5]

INGREDIENTS:

green clay powder	mixed salad ingredients
olive and grapeseed oils	rice or oatcakes
fresh thyme and sage	hummus, cottage cheese
juniper, cardamom and	or free-range eggs
lemon essential oils	natural :
fresh fruits	sunflower seeds
chamomile and	chicken, fish or nut roast
peppermint	fresh vegetables

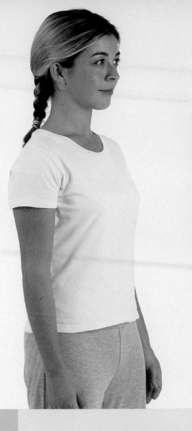

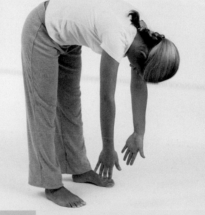

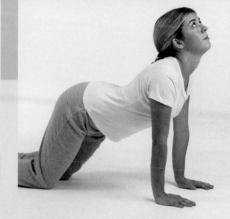

1 Mountain pose: Stand with your feet shoulder-width apart, shoulders relaxed and arms by your sides. Feel your feet firmly on the ground. Breathe deeply, and relax.

2 Standing forward bend: Still standing, lean down slowly until your hands touch the ground. Pause, then slowly ease yourself up again. Repeat 3 times.

3 Cat pose: Kneel on all fours. Relax; then, as you breathe out, arch your back, feeling the stretch all along your spine. Breathe in and release. Repeat 3 times.

4 Child pose: From all fours, rest down on the ground with your arms and feet tucked up underneath you, in a foetal position. Breathe deeply; rest for a few minutes.

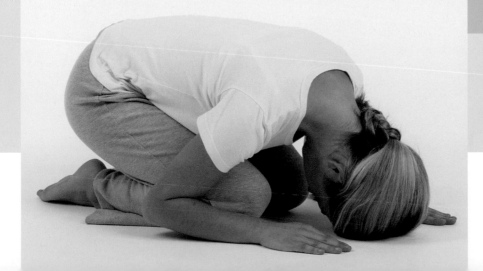

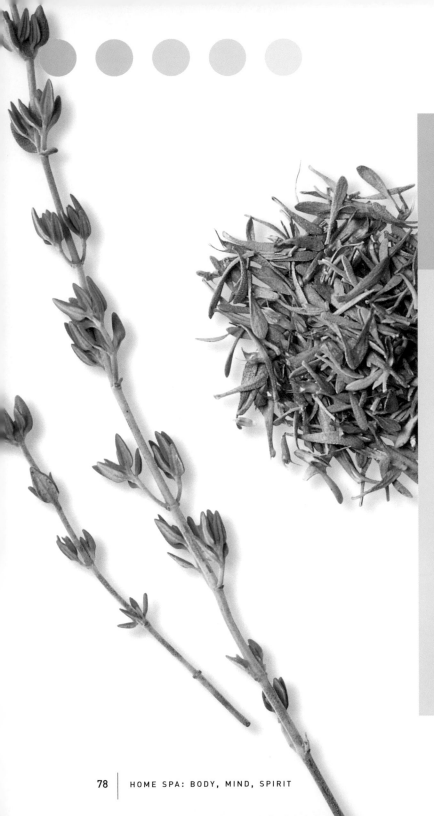

WEEKEND SPA DAY 2 PART 2: DETOXIFYING BODY MASK

After your morning exercise you are going to give each other a body mask, which is an important part of spa treatment. It really targets key areas of the body, such as the waist or thighs, and improves detoxification. It is fun to try at home, but remember that this type of treatment needs preparation and you need all the ingredients and equipment to hand before you begin. Cling film and large towels are important to wrap up the body and increase the heat so that the ingredients can penetrate more effectively. The treatment is best applied and removed in the bathroom; shower it off the skin afterwards. It is best to decide on one particular part of the body to work on, such as the upper back if there are pimples, or the thighs or waist for cellulite or bloating. You will rest with the mask on for 20 minutes; drink water during this time and also after the session.

THYME, SAGE & JUNIPER BODY MASK

This quantity should be enough for both of you.
In a medium-sized bowl put 6 tablespoons green
clay and mix in 180 ml/6 fl oz water to form a paste.
Add 1 tablespoon olive oil and 3 tablespoons fresh
thyme and sage leaves, washed and finely chopped,
and stir into the paste. Then add 6 drops juniper
essential oil, stir again, and the mask is ready to use.
Thyme and sage are skin-cleansing and purifying
herbs, and juniper is one of the best detoxifying
essential oils. Green clay is an excellent purifying
medium, which draws toxins out of the skin, and
olive oil adds nourishment.

MASK APPLICATION

Moisten the skin of the area you want to work on with
a damp flannel, then apply the mask. You will need to
help your partner if she wants it on her back: she
should lie down so that you can spread the mask over
the area, then cover it with a large piece of cling film
and place a towel over that. If you want to work on the
legs, it is easier to apply the mask yourself: just wrap
cling film over the area as above, and wrap in a towel
for 20 minutes. The mask needs to be showered off
thoroughly afterwards. The skin should feel tingly
and glowing.

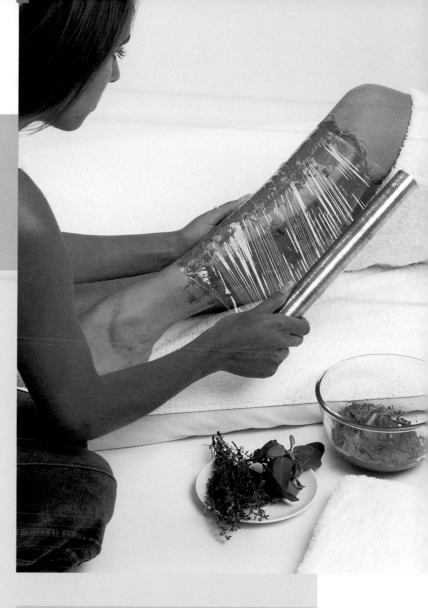

● ● ● ○ **TREATMENT ADVICE**
Use home spa treatments on the day of making.
Avoid contact with the eyes. If the treatment
gets into the eyes, rinse well with warm water.

WEEKEND SPA DAY 2
PART 3: BACK MASSAGE

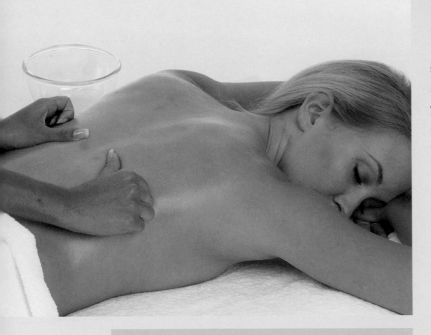

This back massage routine feels really great; it combines sweeping strokes with pressure applied in small circles up either side of the spine. The aromatherapy blend energizes and invigorates, complementing the massage. Make your partner comfortable on the floor on a mat or futon covered with towels; cover her legs and feet to keep them warm while you work. You will be kneeling by her hips on whichever side feels most comfortable.

CARDAMOM, JUNIPER & LEMON BACK MASSAGE BLEND

Pour 4 teaspoons grapeseed oil into a small bowl and add 4 drops cardamom, 4 drops lemon and 2 drops juniper essential oils, which stimulate the circulation. Grapeseed oil is a light massage carrier suitable for all skin types. Stir the blend, then it's ready to use. This quantity will make enough for 2 back massages.

TREATMENT ADVICE

Use home spa treatments on the day of making. Avoid contact with the eyes. If the treatment gets into the eyes, rinse well with warm water.

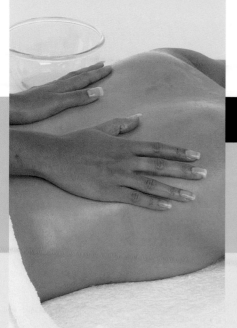

BACK MASSAGE ROUTINE

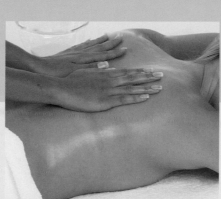

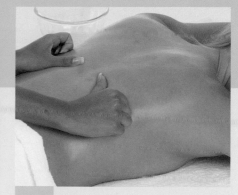

1 Apply 1 teaspoon of the blend to the whole back surface, using fanning movements from the centre out to the sides; make these movements quite brisk as you spread the oil. Add more if you need to, so the skin is well lubricated.

2 With both hands pointing upwards, parallel at the base of the back, stroke slowly up either side of the spine, out across the shoulders and back down the sides. Apply more pressure as you go up and ease off as you come down. Repeat 4 times.

3 Using your thumbs on either side of the spine, starting at the base, apply pressure in rows up towards the shoulders; press for a few seconds then ease off. Repeat this sequence twice.

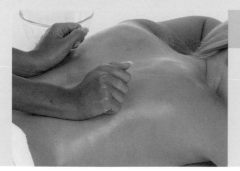

4 With 1 hand on either side of the back, knead your way up the sides and over the shoulders – reverse and come all the way back down again. Keep kneading until you feel that the muscles are loose and relaxed.

5 Repeat the long sweeping strokes of step 2, up and out and down, making the movement slower as you come to the end of the massage. Lift your hands off the back slowly and cover your partner while she rests for a few moments.

WEEKEND SPA DAY 2
PART 4: ENERGY EXERCISE

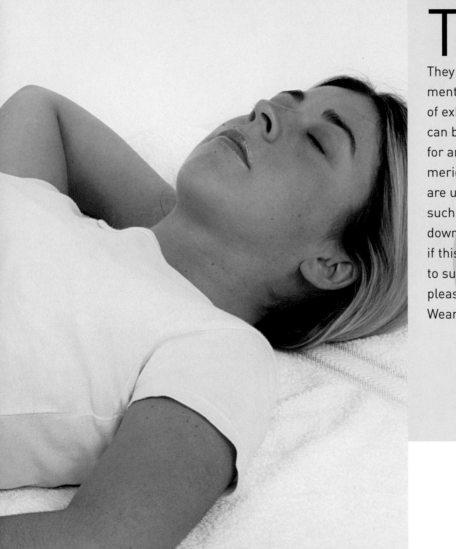

This is a very simple sequence of postures that help to energize and rest the back as well as improve energy levels in the spine. They are very useful for backache, migraines and mental tension, as well as low energy and feelings of exhaustion. You do them by yourself, and they can be used at any time when you feel the need for an energy boost. They have their origin in the meridian-based healing systems of the East, and are used as energy-balancing holds in disciplines such as shiatsu and yoga. You need to be lying down on the floor, preferably completely flat, but if this is very uncomfortable, use a folded towel to support the head. The postures are also very pleasant to enjoy outside, breathing in fresh air. Wear comfortable loose clothes.

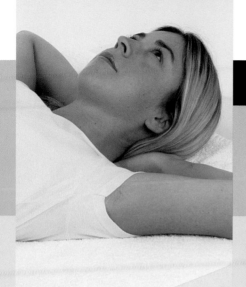

ENERGY EXERCISE

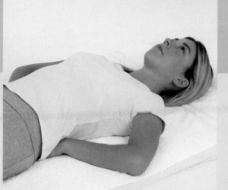

1 Lying flat on your back, simply cradle the base of your skull in your hands. Feel the weight of your head, and let it rest in the support of your fingers. If you like, you can bend your legs and put your feet down flat, to help ease your back at the same time. Stay in the posture for 5 minutes. This posture is very helpful for migraines and neck tension.

2 Lying flat on your back with your legs out straight and your hands palm down, slide your fingers under your lower back where the S-curve of the spine leaves a gap. Your hands should be resting right at the top of your hips. This posture helps to energize the lower back; your hands should begin to feel quite warm. Stay there for 5 minutes; when you want to get up, push down on your hands and use your arms to help you sit up.

3 Lying flat on your back, put your right hand under the base of your skull and your left hand, palm down, at the very base of your spine. Relax, and close your eyes. After a short while you may be able to feel the energy in your spine moving gently between both hands. This is a restful posture, which helps to ease tiredness and low energy.

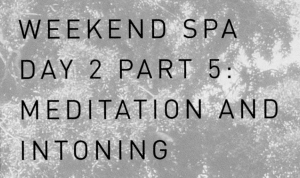

WEEKEND SPA DAY 2 PART 5: MEDITATION AND INTONING

To end your weekend home spa session, here is a meditation and sound exercise to try. This kind of meditation is nothing to do with singing – it is about simple intoning, which is very beneficial to the whole system. Simple sounds, such as 'om', have been chanted for thousands of years; they have a calming and soothing effect on the mind. Use the meditation first, then progress to the intoning. Sit on the floor cross-legged if you are comfortable that way. Otherwise, sit on a hard-backed wooden chair to give you support; both feet should be on the ground, your hands resting in your lap. You might like to record the meditation so that you can listen to the instructions rather than read them.

MEDITATION

Sit relaxed, breathing calmly. Imagine that your toes and feet are becoming like roots, spreading down into the Earth, all the way down as far as they can go. Feel how anchored you are, how the earth supports you. Then imagine that your spine is the trunk of a tree, rising up towards the blue sky, spreading its branches wide towards the sun. Feel yourself perfectly balanced between earth and sky. Breathe in the energy of the sun, imagining it travelling right down to your roots. Then imagine the warm energy of the earth coming back up your roots and into your spine, travelling back up to the sky. This visualization helps you to feel very grounded and balanced.

INTONING

Take a few deep breaths and, at a fairly low, comfortable pitch, intone the sound 'om'. Use up all your breath, then breathe in again, and repeat. Feel how this simple sound resonates inside you, as if you were an empty bowl. As you keep repeating the sound, notice how your body feels. After 6 repetitions, stop intoning and listen to the silence. Breathe easily, and stretch your fingers and toes to finish.

ENDING YOUR WEEKEND SPA

You have spent a weekend eating lightly but nutritiously, exercising and receiving treatments; there has also been time to rest and be quiet. As you

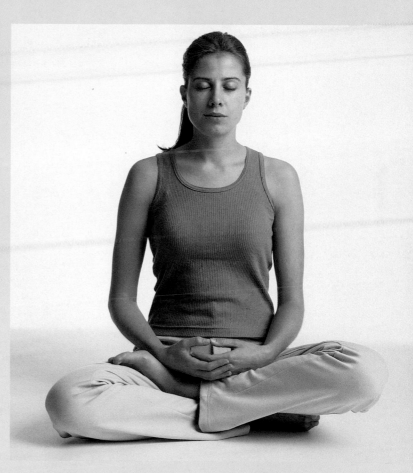

end your home spa weekend, notice how you feel, physically and mentally, and remember how you were when you began. You should feel a big difference. As you resume your everyday life, remember that you can use any individual elements of the home spa routine when you need them to help you de-stress.

CHAPTER FOUR

HOME SPA INGREDIENTS

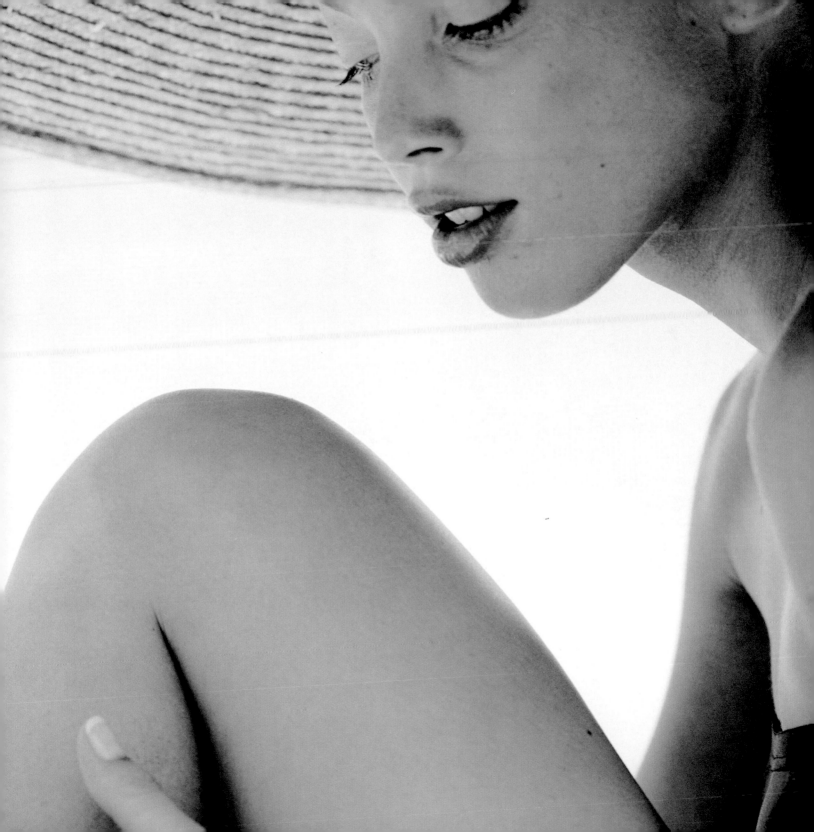

WONDERFUL GIFTS OF NATURE

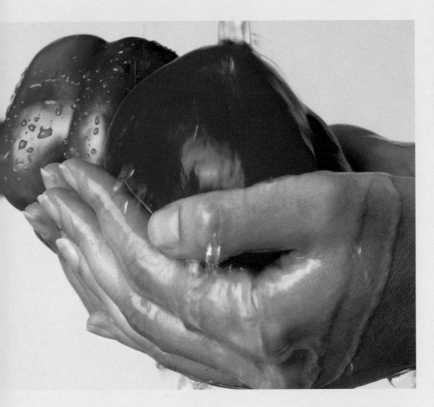

Using totally natural ingredients is a key aspect of the home spa experience. Herbs, essential oils, salts and vegetable carriers – all of these are gently and naturally nourishing and cleansing to the system. Most of the toiletries or face products available on the market are full of artificial chemical preservatives, to which some people are becoming sensitive. Natural ingredients are simple and safe to use, though they do not keep for long periods and must be prepared and used on the same day. You will be amazed at how different your skin feels when it experiences 100 per cent natural and vital skincare – tingling and glowing with health and vitality, soft and supple.

You may already find some of the things you need in your refrigerator or kitchen cupboard; it's surprising how some of the things you eat also function very well as beauty treatments.

USING AND STORING NATURAL INGREDIENTS

Natural ingredients often have a short shelf life, which it is important to observe. Always use these items as fresh as possible in order to get the most benefit from the minerals and vitamins they contain. These benefit your digestion as well as your skin.

Items such as natural yogurt, milk or cream should always be kept refrigerated, and any treatment recipes containing them should be used fresh on the day. Milk should be full cream, as the fat content softens the skin. If you have a dairy allergy, you can use soya milk instead, although the fragrance of the recipe will be affected.

Fruits and vegetables used in recipes should ideally be organic. This is because they are unlikely to have harmful pesticide residues in their skins or flesh. Citrus fruits, for example, have beneficial essential oil in their peel, which is useful in recipes, but the value of the oil would be offset by any chemical residues. All fruit and vegetables must be washed carefully before use.

Essential oils need to be stored in a cool, dark place, with caps tightly closed. Dried herbs need to be stored in glass jars, again ideally in the dark to preserve the active properties of the herb. Fresh herbs can be picked or bought as needed and kept in water for 2 days, then discarded.

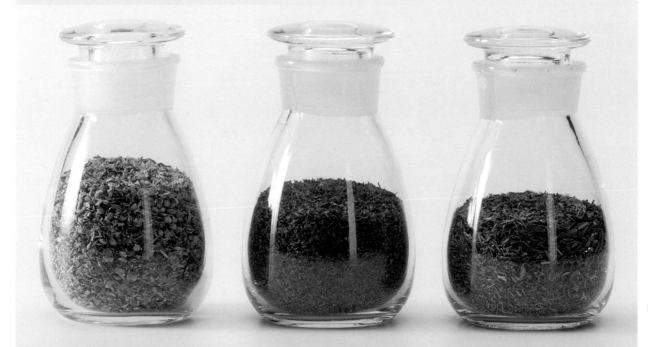

EIGHT HOME SPA ESSENTIAL OILS

Here are the 8 home spa essential oils in more detail. The information here will help you to find out more about the aromatherapy blends that feature in the home spa programmes. Also, the botanical name (in brackets) helps you to purchase the correct essential oil, as some, such as lavender, are produced from different plant species.

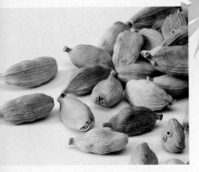

CARDAMOM (Elettaria cardamomum)

Oil obtained from: seeds

Safety check: no issues

Uses: stimulating and warming for poor circulation, aching muscles and sports massage; also relieves backache and stiff neck and shoulders

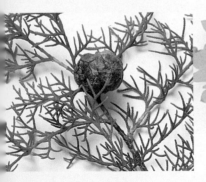

CYPRESS (Cupressus sempervirens)

Oil obtained from: needles and twigs

Safety check: no issues

Uses: skin toning and cleansing for oily and combination skins, detoxifying for cellulite and fluid retention; also helps poor circulation and muscular aches

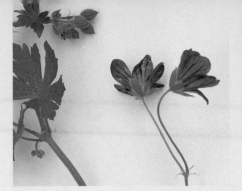

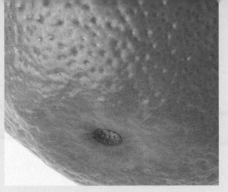

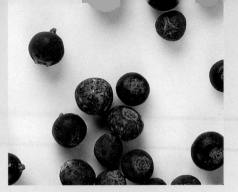

GERANIUM (Pelargonium graveolens)

Oil obtained from: leaves

Safety check: no issues

Uses: balances natural skin oils for all skin types; hydrating and soothing even for sensitive or very dry skin; also helps even out combination skin

GRAPEFRUIT (Citrus paradisi)

Oil obtained from: fruit peel

Safety check: avoid strong UV light on the skin for 12 hours after massage application

Uses: helps detoxify areas of cellulite and fluid retention; useful for cleansing and toning oily or congested skin and removing excess sebum

JUNIPER (Juniperus communis)

Oil obtained from: berries

Safety check: not to be used in pregnancy

Uses: powerfully detoxifying for cellulite and fluid retention; improves the circulation, helps muscular aches; also a good cleanser for oily skin

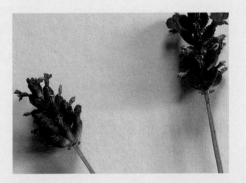

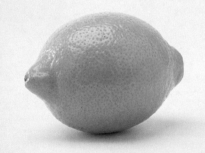

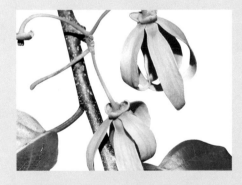

LAVENDER (Lavandula angustifolia)

Oil obtained from: flowers and leaves

Safety check: no issues; can be used neat – 2 drops on a tissue – for acne

Uses: soothing and rejuvenating to all skin types, in cleansers and creams; also relieves muscular aches and headaches

LEMON (Citrus limonum)

Oil obtained from: fruit peel

Safety check: avoid strong UV light on the skin for 12 hours after massage application

Uses: antiseptic and cleansing properties; cleanses greasy or blemished skin; also tones up large pores and improves skin texture

YLANG YLANG (Cananga odorata)

Oil obtained from: flowers

Safety check: no issues

Uses: excellent cleanser for oily skin and hair; balances skin tone and is an excellent treatment for oily congested complexions

EIGHT KEY HOME SPA HERBS

The 8 key home spa herbs can be bought or grown yourself, and used either fresh or dried. Again, the botanical name (in brackets) helps you to identify the correct species to use. Growing your own herbs is very satisfying; you can then use them for health purposes as well as for flavouring food.

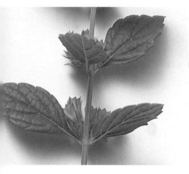

MELISSA (Melissa officinalis)

Part used: leaves

Safety check: no issues

Uses: skin calming and restorative in baths, foot baths and facial steams; a cool infusion calms irritated skin; a hot infusion helps headaches or indigestion

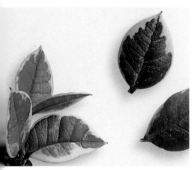

MYRTLE (Myrtus communis)

Part used: leaves or flowers

Safety check: no issues

Uses: refreshing and toning to the skin; the leaves are more clarifying, in the bath as well as on the face; a cool infusion of flowers soothes the skin; a hot leaf infusion is a refreshing digestive tonic

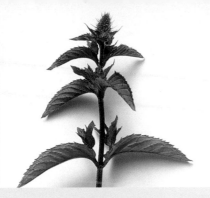

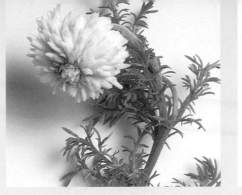

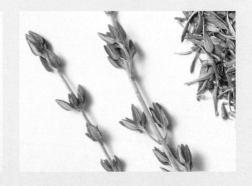

PEPPERMINT (Mentha x piperita)

Part used: leaves

Safety check: no issues

Uses: fresh and invigorating in baths, foot baths, facial steams and cleansing masks; the menthol content deodorizes the feet; an infusion helps indigestion

ROMAN CHAMOMILE (Anthemis nobilis)

Part used: flowers

Safety check: no issues

Uses: soothing and anti-inflammatory for dry and sensitive skins; excellent in facial steams and baths to cleanse the skin gently; an infusion eases headaches and stress

ROSEMARY (Rosmarinus officinalis)

Part used: leaves

Safety check: drinking rosemary infusions is not recommended in pregnancy

Uses: warms stiff muscles, especially in the bath or in foot baths; also eases pain in the joints; an infusion is a very good scalp and hair tonic

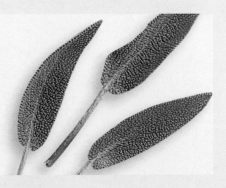

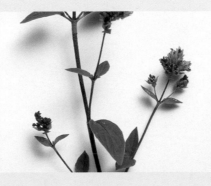

SAGE (Salvia officinalis)

Part used: leaves

Safety check: use in moderation as it has a strong effect

Uses: toning and powerfully cleansing in baths, foot baths and detoxifying skin treatments; improves the circulation and warms stiff limbs, as well as cleansing the skin

SWEET MARJORAM (Origanum marjorana)

Part used: leaves

Safety check: no issues

Uses: soothes the joints and eases muscular aches and pains, in baths or foot baths, particularly in the evening; also helps with poor sleep, soothes stress and calms indigestion

THYME (Thymus vulgaris)

Part used: leaves

Safety check: no issues

Uses: encourages sweating, so is useful in a detoxifying Epsom salts bath, where it eases aches and pains and soothes the joints; a foot bath helps aching feet

HOME SPA SALTS

Salts are a vital part of the spa experience. Sea bathing has been used as a health treatment for centuries: the salt water tones the circulation, encourages detoxification and smooths the skin. A daily dip in the sea was considered to be a major health tonic by the Ancient Greek father of modern medicine, Hippocrates. Different salts are used for different purposes in spa treatment.

DEAD SEA MINERAL SALTS

These are special salts from the Dead Sea in Israel. The water is so impregnated with minerals that if you swim there it is virtually impossible to sink. High levels of potassium, sodium and magnesium make Dead Sea salts very detoxifying; hospitals in Israel offer salt treatments for rheumatism and arthritis. The minerals are also skin soothing and rejuvenating and have been used in soaps, lotions and creams for centuries. After a Dead Sea salt bath, your skin will feel incredibly smooth and soft.

Epsom salts

This is a mineral salt with a very high magnesium content. Its effect is invigorating, encouraging the pores to open and allowing the skin to rid itself of impurities. After an Epsom salts bath, you will find that you continue to sweat, so it is important to keep yourself very warm; you may find you want to shower later. Epsom salts baths are also good for aches and pains, or after gardening.

Sea salt

Look for good quality salt from a single geographical source, such as the south of France. Sea salt comes in fine and coarse grains; for body and face scrubs, the finer grains have a less abrasive effect. Sea salt is invigorating as a treatment ingredient, stimulating local circulation and making the skin glow. Use it as a scrub in the bath or shower, or dissolve 4 tablespoons sea salt in a hot bath as a cleansing treatment, adding 2 tablespoons sage or thyme for their cleansing properties.

Seaweed

In the professional spa world, seaweeds are well-known sources of essential minerals and vitamins that assist the process of detoxification. Seaweed masks, body wraps and packs are used for deep cleansing and even weight loss. It is not easy to prepare seaweed treatments yourself at home, but you can supplement your home spa routine with quality seaweed-based body and skin products from good retail outlets.

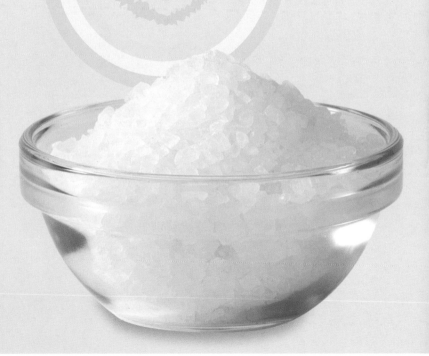

HOME SPA CLEANSERS AND EXFOLIATORS

Cleansing and exfoliating are very important processes in a spa context. Cleansing means lifting dirt and impurities out of the skin, and exfoliating means using a more abrasive ingredient to gently rub dead cells off the surface of the skin to brighten the complexion and stimulate new cell growth. Both are needed to give the skin a really deep treatment. Natural ingredients help both cleansing and exfoliating to happen gently, without the need for harsh chemicals.

CLEANSERS

GREEN CLAY

This is a superb deep cleanser, used for making masks. It is full of minerals that detoxify the skin and also have anti-inflammatory effects. Green clay gently draws out impurities from the skin and helps to treat blemishes

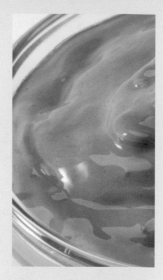

HONEY

Used as a cleanser for centuries, honey is cleansing and antiseptic. Honey in face masks and cleansers helps blemished skin by preventing scarring. Use honey from a single source and try to ensure that it has not been heat-treated or blended – this destroys its active vitamin and mineral content

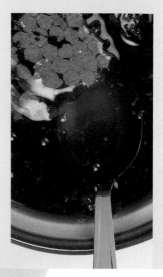

EXFOLIATORS

MILK

Whisk equal parts of chamomile or myrtle infusion with full cream milk to make a nourishing skin cleanser. Milk is high in protein, calcium and other minerals that make the skin soft and supple; milk baths soothe the skin. If you have a dairy allergy you can try using soya milk, but the properties are not as nourishing

NATURAL YOGURT

Natural yogurt is an excellent cooling and hydrating cleanser and can be used on all skin types; it also makes a simple and effective face mask. It is slightly acid, so it protects the upper skin layers from harmful bacteria

GRANULATED SUGAR

This has a long history of use, particularly in the Middle East. It exfoliates the skin gently and is good in body scrubs, blended with different crushed fruits

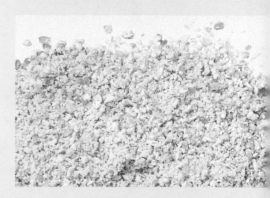

OATMEAL

Oats have traditionally been used for softening the skin and removing impurities; they also have an anti-inflammatory effect. Fine oatmeal is best for skin pastes, which gently cleanse and soothe

GROUND ALMONDS

The finely ground nuts polish and smooth the complexion, helping to nourish dry skin and eliminate blemishes. Ground almonds make good face pastes for exfoliating dry or mature skin

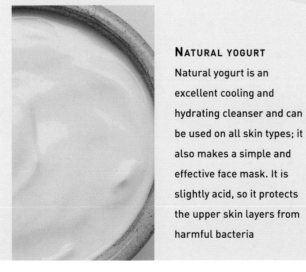

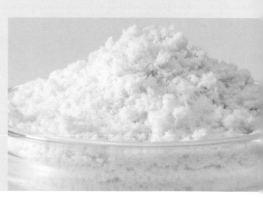

HOME SPA TONERS
AND SKIN SOOTHERS

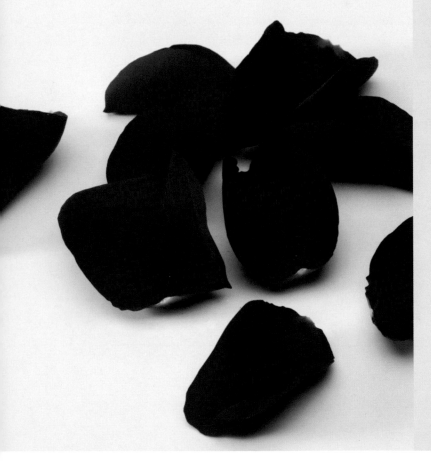

After cleansing, it is important to tone the skin using a water-based product. This removes any last traces of cleanser, as well as freshening and hydrating the skin. Toners also help to close up large pores and improve the surface texture. Many commercial toners contain alcohol, which can dry the skin, so it's good to know that there are natural alternatives that work gently and efficiently. These products need to be refrigerated and used up while they are fresh (within 3 months in the case of flower waters). Aloe vera gel also features here as one of the best natural skin soothers.

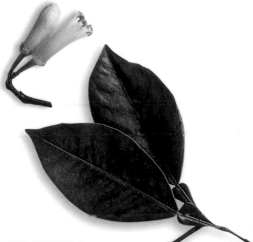

FLOWER WATERS

ORANGE FLOWER WATER This is a by-product of the distillation process that produces orange blossom (neroli) essential oil. Exquisitely perfumed, it contains minute traces of the oil. It soothes and nourishes dry and mature skins, and also gently cleanses oily or combination skins. It is particularly refreshing to use after a deep cleansing face pack. Avoid contact with the eyes. If the product gets into the eyes, rinse well with warm water.

ROSE WATER True rose water is a distillation water from the production of rose essential oil. The water is the medium in which the flower petals are soaked before being heated; it contains minute traces of essential oil from the petals. Rose water has been used for centuries as a skin cooling and soothing lotion. Use it to tone and soothe dry, sensitive or mature skin. Avoid contact with the eyes. If the product gets into the eyes, rinse well with warm water.

NB: Both these flower waters need to be kept in the refrigerator and used up within 3 months.

HERBAL INFUSIONS

These are toners you can make up yourself. Simply make the herbal tea using 1 teaspoon dried herb or 2 teaspoons fresh herb to 120 ml/4 fl oz boiling water, then infuse for 15 minutes, strain and pour into a clean glass bottle. Refrigerate and use over 2 days. Avoid contact with the eyes. If the product gets into the eyes, rinse well with warm water.

CHAMOMILE calms and soothes irritated or sensitive skin

LAVENDER FLOWER soothes and tones oily or combination skin

MYRTLE LEAF refreshes and tones all skin types

SUPER SKIN SOOTHER

ALOE VERA GEL Aloe vera gel is a wonderful natural product that instantly cools red, itching or sunburnt skin. Aloe vera leaves contain the juice that is made into the gel. In Jamaica, the leaves are simply picked and the liquid applied instantly to damaged skin. It is possible to buy quality aloe vera gel from health food stores; keep refrigerated and use up according to the manufacturer's guidelines

HOME SPA
CARRIER OILS

These quality fruit and vegetable oils are the best way of nourishing the skin, as well as being the medium for carrying essential oils from aromatherapy blends straight into the skin layers. When buying carrier oils, look for organic cold-pressed oils; these contain the maximum quantities of fat-soluble vitamins, which are the food your skin truly needs. During a home spa it is good to treat your body and face to these oils and let your skin absorb the benefits.

APRICOT KERNEL (Prunus armeniaca)
The seed of the apricot yields this excellent light carrier, which is very useful for face massage. It is rich in fatty acids, which nourish the upper skin layers and encourage a smooth and soft complexion. Apricot kernel is particularly good for dry, sensitive or mature skins

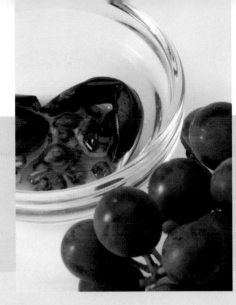

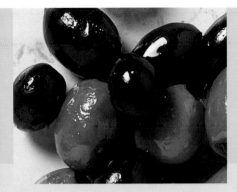

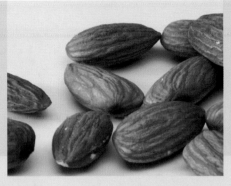

GRAPESEED (Vitis vinifera)

The seeds from grapes yield a light green carrier oil that is one of the best for body massage, particularly if your skin is already quite supple. It is also good for massaging blemished skin because it leaves very little residue. The end result is skin with a silky soft surface

JOJOBA (Simmondsia chinensis)

This wonderful golden liquid is, in fact, a wax, so it would go solid if kept in the refigerator. Keep it instead in a cool, dark place. Jojoba has the advantage of being very similar to the skin's own lubricating oils. It works very well as an oil cleanser for the face, as it dissolves dirt out of the pores. It also performs excellently as a nourishing body massage oil

OLIVE (Olea europea)

This is a wonderful skin lubricant with centuries of use behind it. Extra virgin olive oil is best for spa work because of the high vitamin and mineral content. It already has a distinctive aroma, and so does not work as an aromatherapy base; however, it is extremely good in body scrubs and hair wraps as an excellent nourishing ingredient. It is rich in vitamin E, which is an excellent antioxidant, therefore helping to protect skin and hair from environmental damage

SWEET ALMOND
(Prunus amygdalus var. dulcis)

This carrier is pressed from sweet almond nuts, which, in the form of ground almonds, can also be used as a nourishing and exfoliating skin paste. Sweet almond oil contains fatty acids, which help to encourage healthy skin, hair and nails. It is very useful in body and face massage, and is especially good for dry skins

CHAPTER FIVE

SPA FOR LIFE

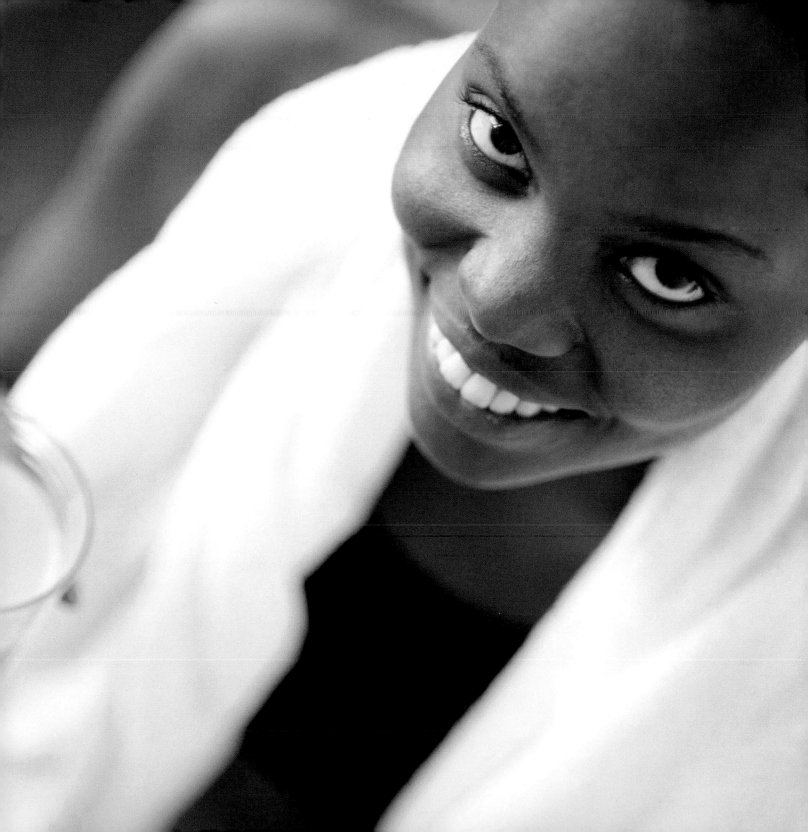

WHEN TO ENJOY A SPA

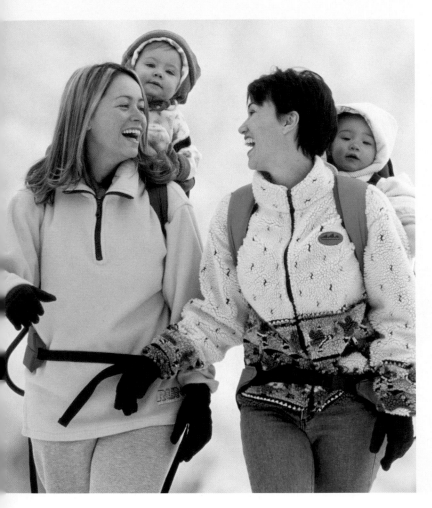

Now that you have explored so many different aspects of the home spa, it is useful to think about bringing these health-giving techniques into your life on a regular basis. Although a one-off experience is very pleasant, it cannot contribute to your overall health and well-being in the long term. In continental Europe, the spa tradition is taken seriously, and people make regular visits to their spa. Spa techniques can build your health and energy, and they are best enjoyed over a period of time. Looking at the year, here are some ideas to show how a spa could help you.

WINTER

This is usually a time of less physical activity and possibly less time outside. A home spa will encourage you to go out into the bracing fresh air and clear your lungs. At a time when immune infections are around, deep cleansing spa techniques and massage with essential oils help to boost your immunity so that you stay fit and well. Even if the weather outside is cold, you can enjoy home spa massages indoors.

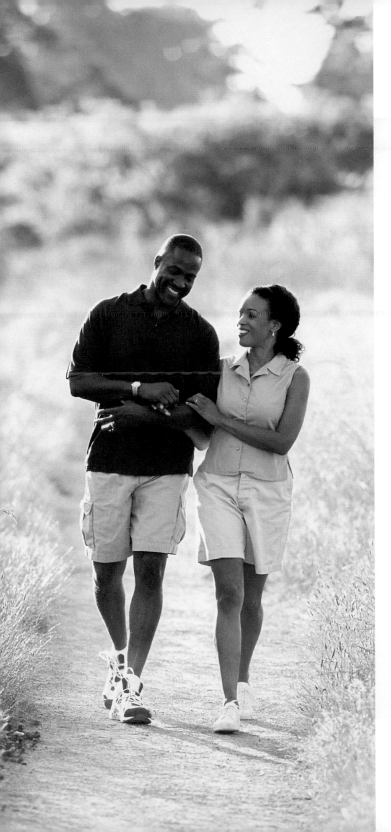

SPRING

As nature wakes up in the springtime, so does your body; home spa techniques can help you to detoxify by stimulating blood circulation and building up your energy levels. Using body masks and scrubs will exfoliate your skin and remove dead cells, leaving you revitalized and refreshed. You will feel encouraged to get out and enjoy the lighter days of spring.

SUMMER

When all the summer fruits are in season, now is a great time to enjoy a cleansing diet as well as pamper your skin with deeply nourishing carrier oils, masks and massage. The skin is more exposed during the summertime, and therefore more prone to dryness. Using a home spa helps you take advantage of all the opportunities summer brings to enjoy the outdoors and cleanse your whole system.

AUTUMN

As the days draw in, there are still wonderful sights and colours to be enjoyed outdoors. Use aromatherapy and herb treatments to tone and energize your body. Autumn can be a challenging transition, with mood changes as the days get shorter; immune infections can already occur. Stay bright and uplifted with home spa techniques to cleanse and refresh your whole system.

CREATING YOUR
OWN HOME SPA ROUTINES

In addition to using the suggested formats in this book, you can, of course, pick and choose different treatments and recipes and combine them as you like to create your own individual home spa routines. You may have certain preferences for treatment, such as more massage or facial work; you may want to increase the exercise time or vary the meditations. This is absolutely fine, and in fact it makes the home spa experience all the more personal. It just takes a bit more planning to make sure you have time to fit it all in. It's surprising how long it can take to get things ready, which is why the routines in this book are well spaced out to allow time for preparation.

As a guide to creating your own routines, think about what you want to achieve with the home spa. Is it to detoxify, to deeply cleanse the skin or to relax? Is it to work on a particular body area that needs attention? Will you be working on your own or will there be someone else sharing the spa with you? Once you

have that focus, you can use this book to select the treatments and recipes you will need.

You can use a one- or two-day home spa once a month to help yourself rest, relax and re-energize your batteries. In fact, this is one of the best treats you can give your whole system. If you build it into your regular routine, you will find many knock-on benefits – such as quality sleep, better digestion and improved energy levels.

Through regular home spa routines you will become more aware of how your mental and physical health are interlinked. You will notice the effects your lifestyle has on your system, and you will have the tools to correct imbalances. Increasing your own personal awareness of mental and physical balance will help you to achieve renewed strength and energy. As the Ancient Greeks believed, a healthy mind in a healthy body is the best recipe for life. Enjoy your spa sessions, and have fun looking after your body.

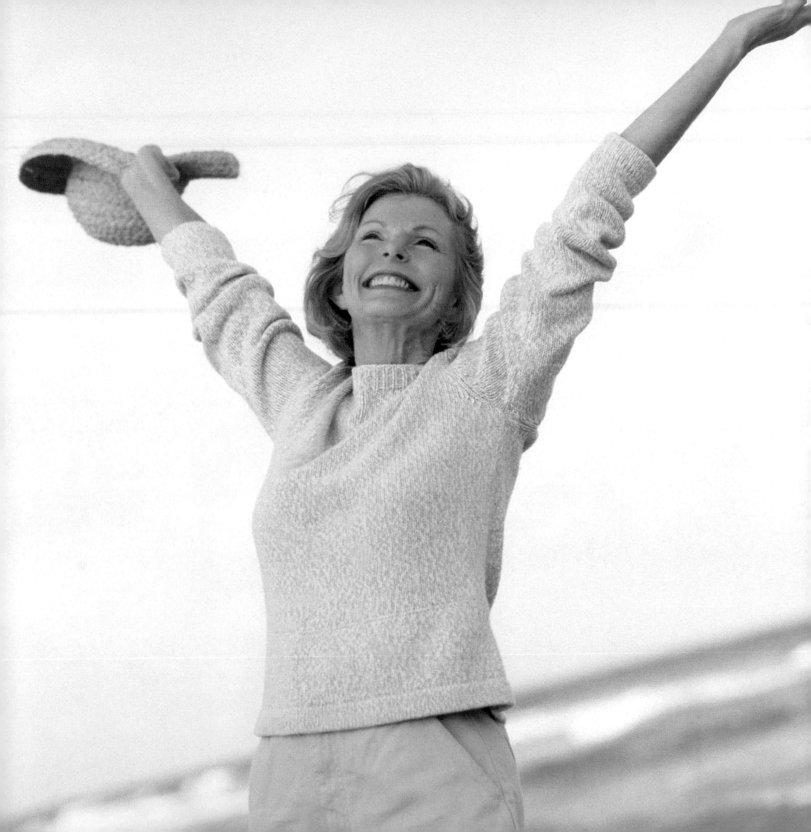

GLOSSARY

ACUPRESSURE: a system of using pressure points along specific pathways in the body to stimulate the meridians (the main energy channels in Chinese medicine)

ANTI-INFLAMMATORY: a substance that reduces inflammation

AROMATHERAPY: applying natural fragrances – essential oils – to the body in various ways

BODY THERAPY: various massage treatments designed to ease out physical tensions and assist repair

CARRIER OIL: a vegetable oil used for dissolving essential oils in aromatherapy blends

DETOXIFYING: an action that helps the elimination of toxins from the system, usually via the kidneys

DIETARY THERAPY: a spa therapy in which particular foods and drinks are provided to cleanse the system from inside

DRAINAGE: name given to massage movements in which strokes work up towards the heart, encouraging excess fluid out of the body

ESSENTIAL OIL: a liquid natural fragrance extracted from a single plant source

EXFOLIATION: a process that removes loose dead skin cells from the skin surface

HYDRATING: a substance that adds moisture when applied to the skin

HYDROTHERAPY: various spa techniques involving water for cleansing and detoxification

INFUSION: a herb soaked in boiling water (tea)

KNEADING: a massage stroke in which the muscles are squeezed like dough

PRESSURE STROKES: a massage technique for applying pressure on a small area of the body using thumbs or individual fingers

SEBUM: the skin's own natural lubricant

TONING: an action that tightens up slack skin

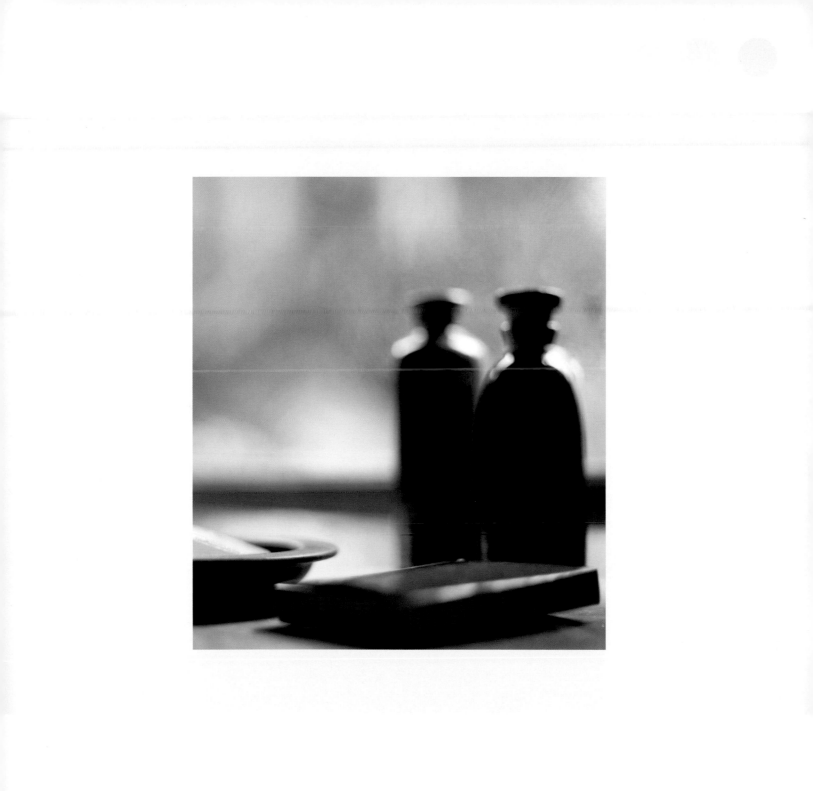

INDEX

INDEX

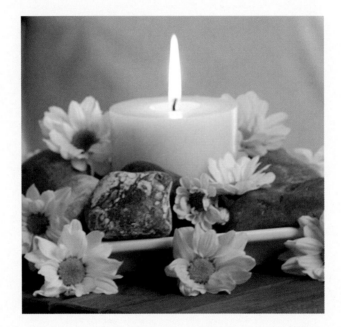